THE ART OF AGING

Embracing Life in Your Golden Years

Dr. Suzanne Alari

Table of Contents

INTRODUCTION

As a medical doctor with twenty years of experience, I have treated and assisted many patients through aging. Having lived through the physical and emotional changes of aging and witnessed my mother's transition from a vibrant woman in her youth to a frail elder, I understand the aging process's unique challenges. These events have taught me that growing old is not the final step towards the grave but rather a time to embrace life and the opportunities it presents. When it comes to aging, our society greatly emphasizes negative aspects such as wrinkles, memory loss, and physical limitations. However, much more positives to growing old should be discussed.

Through this book, I will provide you with insight into the many positive aspects of aging. In The Art of Aging, I will share my experience, knowledge, and tips on making the most of your golden years. I will help you discover how to enjoy life and experience new adventures in retirement. You will learn how to stay physically and mentally healthy and find joy in the simple things.

I will also discuss the importance of maintaining relationships with friends and family and staying connected with the world around you.

The Art of Aging is a guide to help you embrace life in your golden years.

I hope you will find this book informative, engaging, and inspiring.

If you make the most of your retirement, you will live a more meaningful life. So let's begin this journey and explore the art of aging together!

CHAPTER 1

UNDERSTANDING THE PROCESS OF AGING

Understanding the aging process can be a difficult and emotional experience, especially for those nearing retirement. The fear of the future, being alone, and coming to terms with one's own mortality can be overwhelming. It can be tough when a person takes stock of their life and finds it wanting, feeling that they have made no meaningful impact. Loss of independence can also be difficult to accept at one age.

It is natural for our bodies to undergo changes as we age. These changes can range from noticeable physical changes to more subtle changes such as mood swings, cognitive decline, and changes in ability.

This chapter will discuss the physical, mental, emotional, social, and spiritual changes that occur as we age and how to manage them.

PHYSICAL CHANGES IN AGING

Let's start by discussing the physical changes in aging; one of the most obvious physical changes is decreased mobility. Our muscles and joints become stiffer, and it takes longer to complete physical activities. This can be especially noticeable in our legs, back, and neck. This forms part of a natural wear-and-tear process that affects the ligaments and cartilage in our joints. Osteoarthritis, inflammatory conditions (Bursitis, tendonitis & gout), and autoimmune conditions like Rheumatoid arthritis can also affect our mobility and quality of life.

In addition, our bones become weaker, making us more susceptible to fractures and other injuries. This is caused by a natural decline in the bone mineral density (BMD). The most common factors contributing to this decline are the reduction in physical activity, a poor diet that is low in Vit D and Calcium, to name a few, and the presence of certain chronic medications. Women are also affected by the gradual decline of estrogen during menopause. As a result, it is important to stay active and ensure that you have a balanced diet to limit the decline in bone density.

Another physical change that comes with aging is decreased vision and hearing. Our eyesight may become blurred, or we may develop cataracts, making it harder to see clearly. These are due to changes in proteins in the lens of the eye as well as the elasticity of the lens. Other factors affecting vision are decreased blood flow to the retina or increased pressure in the eye (Glaucoma).

Our hearing may also become impaired, making it difficult to hear conversations or to pick up on high-pitched noises (Presbyopia). Exposure to loud noises during your life will also damage the inner ear and lead to a loss of hearing in old age. Visiting your doctor for regular eye and ear exams is important to catch any changes early.

As we age, our skin also changes. This can include wrinkles, age spots, thinning skin, and dryness. Skin elasticity decreases, making it harder for our skin to bounce back after stretching. This can lead to sagging skin and a decrease in the natural glow of our skin. This can be attributed to the reduction of collagen in our skin over time. Other factors like smoking, regular and prolonged sun (UV) exposure, or dehydration can also affect our skin's elasticity, leading to deeper wrinkles.

It is good you practice good skin care and use moisturizers and sunscreen to help protect your skin from a young age. It will lessen the effects of damage to the skin in later life.

Finally, our immune system weakens, making us more susceptible to illness and disease. This is due to a decrease in T-cells and B-cells in our bodies. These are cells that help fight infections and produce antibodies. Stress and chronic inflammation are two important factors that we have only started to come to grips with over the past few decades. Their effect on the immune system is immense and has been mostly overlooked in the past century.

It is, therefore, important to boost your immune system. This includes exercising regularly, eating a balanced diet, getting enough sleep, and avoiding stress (which is easier said than done in today's modern age).

These physical changes can be daunting, but with the right attitude and lifestyle, you can still live an active and healthy life in your golden years. By recognizing and addressing the physical changes that come with aging, you can ensure that you continue to live life to the fullest.

As a medical doctor that has cared for the aged, I have helped many make important health decisions. I have worked with them to promote healthy aging by encouraging them to stay active and eat a balanced diet. I have also helped them maintain their strength and mobility by assisting them in finding safe and effective exercises for their age. Additionally, I have assisted in exploring options for preserving their vision, hearing, and other senses.

I was also a great source of emotional support for my mother. I try to provide her with an outlet for her feelings and help her to navigate the changes that come with aging. Ultimately, my goal is to ensure that the physical and emotional needs of the aged are met and that they can age gracefully. I hope you also make the most of your golden years through my guidance and support.

MENTAL AND EMOTIONAL CHANGES IN AGING

While physical changes are well known, mental and emotional changes are less discussed. This chapter will discuss the mental and emotional changes that occur during aging.

The mental changes aging process can bring about changes in mental abilities. These changes can range from mild to severe, depending on the individual. One of the most common mental changes associated with aging is memory decline.

As we age, our memory becomes less reliable, and we forget things more easily. In addition, our ability to process new information decreases, and our reaction time slows down.

Aging also affects our ability to make decisions. Our ability to think logically and evaluate information decreases, making it harder to make decisions. We may also become more easily confused or overwhelmed. Another common mental change is increased difficulty in problem-solving. It takes longer to work through a problem and develop solutions with age.

In addition to mental changes, the aged also undergo emotional changes. One of the most common emotional changes associated with aging is decreased self-confidence. As we age, we may start to feel less capable or competent. This can lead to feelings of insecurity, fear, and anxiety.

Aging can also lead to increased emotional sensitivity. We may become more easily overwhelmed or overwhelmed by our emotions. We may also become more easily frustrated or agitated.

Aging can also lead to an increased sense of loneliness. We may feel isolated and disconnected from friends and family, leading to sadness and depression.

It is essential to recognize these changes and take steps to manage them. With the right support and tools, it is possible to cope with the mental and emotional changes of aging and enjoy a fulfilling life.

SOCIAL CHANGES IN AGING

Our social circles can often shrink as we age - but why does this happen? It could be due to various factors, from physical to life changes. Physical changes can be a major cause of a shrinking social circle. As we age, our physical abilities can start to decline, making it harder to participate in activities we used to enjoy. This can make it challenging to maintain friendships, as we may no longer be able to do the things we used to with our friends.

Additionally, our physical health can start to decline, making it harder to maintain contact with friends. Life changes can also cause a shrinking social circle. As we age, we may move to a new location, or our lives may drastically change due to different life events such as marriage, children, or retirement. In these cases, our old friends may be unable to keep up with us due to their own life changes, so we can no longer maintain contact.

Loss of social contact can also be caused by death. As we grow older, our friends and family members may start to pass away, leaving us without the social contacts we once had. This can be especially difficult to cope with, as it can make us feel isolated and alone. The good news is a shrinking social circle doesn't have to be permanent. Even as we age, various ways exist to expand our social circles. We can join clubs or groups that focus on activities we're interested in or look for online communities to connect with people who share similar interests.

Additionally, we can use social media or dating apps to connect with others or even to reconnect with old friends. Although aging can lead to a shrinking social circle, it doesn't have to be permanent. With the proper steps, we can expand our social circles and stay in touch with friends and family.

SPIRITUAL CHANGES IN AGING

The aging process is an inevitable part of life; for many, it is accompanied by a range of spiritual changes.

As we age, our views of the world and our place in it often shift, which can profoundly impact our spiritual well-being. One of the most common spiritual changes that come with aging is the realization of mortality. As we age, we become more aware of our own mortality and the fact that our lives are finite.

This can be a difficult reality, especially for those with strong religious beliefs. For those who believe in an afterlife, this can be a source of comfort, but for those who don't, it can be a source of fear and anxiety.

The idea of mortality can also bring about a sense of acceptance and appreciation for life. As we age, we become more aware of how precious life is and how quickly it can pass. As a result, we might feel more grateful for our time and motivated to use it wisely. Also, it can cause us to feel more appreciative of the people and experiences we have in life and a stronger desire to hold onto them.

Aging can also bring about a greater sense of self-awareness. As we age, we become more aware of our strengths and weaknesses and how we fit into the world. This can lead to a greater understanding of our purpose in life and a desire to live life to the fullest.

For some, aging can bring about a greater sense of spiritual connection. As we become older, we frequently realize more about how interrelated all life is and how important each of us is to the overall scheme of things. This can lead to a sense of spiritual connectedness, bringing great comfort and peace. As we age, we may also find ourselves struggling with the idea of death and dying. We may find ourselves struggling to accept the inevitability of our own death and the death of those we love. This can be a difficult and painful process but can also lead to a greater sense of peace and understanding.

The spiritual changes that come with aging are often uncomfortable and difficult to accept, but they can also be a source of great insight and growth. As we age, we can use these changes to deepen our understanding of ourselves and our place in the world. These changes can lead to greater peace and contentment with time and patience.

CHAPTER 2

THE PHYSICAL CHANGES OF AGING – HOW TO OVERCOME AND LIMIT THEIR EFFECT

The physical changes of aging can be a difficult thing to deal with for many people. As our bodies start to age, these physical changes we experience can be difficult to cope with, both emotionally and physically. As said in the previous chapter, these changes can range from wrinkles and gray hair to joint pain and decreased mobility. While it may seem like these changes are inevitable, there are ways to limit their effects and even overcome them in some cases.

In this chapter, we'll look at the physical changes of aging, how they can affect us, and how we can limit and even overcome their effects.

First, what causes aging? Before we can talk about the physical changes of aging, it's important to understand what causes aging in the first place.

I was as naive as many of the younger generation today when I first noticed my mother's age catching up to her. I remember coming home on different occasions and seeing her walking more slowly than usual.

She was my rock, my champion, and I had never seen her look so fragile. As time passed, I noticed more and more signs that my mother was aging. She would become tired easily and often needed to rest. She often forgot things, like where she left her keys or what she talked about mid-conversation. I couldn't bear to see her like this, and I found myself wishing that things could return to how they used to be.

I resolved to take matters into my own hands and began to do whatever I could to help my mother. I took over more household chores and tried my best to make her life easier. I also began taking on a more nurturing role in our relationship, giving her hugs and cuddles whenever needed. I also tried to stay positive and celebrate the little moments. I would remind my mother of everything she had accomplished over the years and our shared memories. I wanted her to know that no matter how old she got, she would always be my mother, and I would always love her.

My mother's age and frailty were natural, but I was resolved to make the best of it. I'm so thankful for all the time I spent with her, even if it was more difficult than before. Despite having to see her get older, I will always treasure the memories we shared. Aging is caused by a combination of factors, including genetics, lifestyle, and environmental factors. Genetics is the most important factor in determining how quickly a person will age. It plays a major role in determining how quickly our bodies degenerate over time.

The way a person lives has a big impact on how quickly they age. A good diet, regular exercise, and sufficient rest contribute to a slower aging process. Environmental factors, such as pollution and sun exposure, can also impact how quickly a person ages. The skin can age prematurely due to exposure to contaminants like cigarette smoke and UV radiation.

Now that we understand what causes aging let's look at some common physical aging changes. One of the most common physical changes of aging is wrinkles.

Wrinkles are caused by a breakdown of the skin's collagen and elastin, which leads to sagging and lines on the skin.

Gray hair is another common physical change of aging. As we age, our bodies produce less pigment that gives our hair its color, leading to gray hair.

Joint pain is also a common physical change of aging. As we age, our joints are subject to wear and tear from years of use. This can cause joints to become stiffer and less mobile, and muscles can become weaker and more prone to injury. Our bodies produce less natural lubrication for our joints, making them less flexible and more prone to injury. Also, our bones and muscles can become less dense, making them more prone to injury and less able to support our bodies. Inflammation can cause pain and stiffness in our joints, making them less flexible. It becomes more challenging to move our joints when we have arthritis, a common ailment that can cause discomfort, stiffness, and swelling in the joints. All of these reduce our body's suppleness.

The first step in limiting the effects of aging is to lead a healthy lifestyle.

It's crucial to consume a nutritious diet, exercise frequently, and get enough sleep to slow down the aging process. In addition to leading a healthy lifestyle, protecting the skin from environmental factors is crucial for limiting aging effects. Wearing sunscreen and avoiding smoking and excessive sun exposure can help protect the skin from premature aging.

Let's look at the following in more detail:

i. Exercise and Physical activities (ii) Nutrition and Diet (iii) Benefits of Maintaining good hygiene (iv) Benefits of getting enough sleep

EXERCISE AND PHYSICAL ACTIVITIES

Exercise and physical activity are two of the most important factors for a healthy life. Physical activity is the best way to keep our bodies strong and energetic as we age, which is why it is vital.

Not only does exercise help to keep us fit and strong, but it can also help to limit the effects of aging on the elderly. Exercise can help to reduce inflammation, help maintain muscle mass, improve cardiovascular health, increase bone density, improve overall health, reduce the risk of diseases such as heart disease, stroke, and diabetes, and even help slow down the aging process.

Exercise helps reduce inflammation in the body by helping to reduce oxidative stress, which can damage cells and lead to a wide range of illnesses.

As you get older, you tend to lose muscle mass. Regular exercise can help maintain muscle mass, which helps keep the body strong and functional.

It helps improve cardiovascular health by strengthening the heart and improving circulation, lower blood pressure, reducing cholesterol levels, and the risk of stroke or heart attack.

It also helps increase bone density, which helps reduce the risk of fractures and osteoporosis. Exercises involving weight, including jogging, lifting weights, and walking, are particularly helpful for boosting bone density.

This chapter is also written to explore the different ways that exercise and physical activity can help to overcome and limit the effects of aging on the elderly.

Benefits of Exercise for the Elderly

Exercise is beneficial for all age groups, but it is especially important for the elderly.

Frequent exercise can enhance physical health, lower injury risk, and lower the risk of developing age-related disorders. It can also help to improve mental health and can even improve mood, and help to reduce stress and anxiety.

Enhancing balance and coordination through exercise can assist in lowering the chance of falling. In addition to lowering the risk of falling and enhancing general physical health, exercise can help to improve cardiovascular fitness and muscle strength.

Exercise can also aid in lowering the risk of age-related illnesses like diabetes, heart disease, and stroke. Regular physical activity can help improve blood pressure, cholesterol, and blood sugar levels. Also, it can aid in lowering the chance of developing some cancers, including breast and colon cancer.

Exercise can also help to prevent and manage osteoporosis, and it can help to improve sleep quality.

Exercise and Physical Activity for the Elderly

As you age, you need to find an exercise routine that works for you.

I recommend low-impact activities such as walking, swimming, yoga, and Tai Chi, as they are all good options for you as you age.

Strength training is also important for you, as it can help to improve muscle strength and balance. It would help if you also focused on balance and flexibility exercises, such as balance boards and stretching. Balance exercises can help to reduce the risk of falls, and flexibility exercises can help to improve mobility and range of motion. The elderly should also drink plenty of water and get enough sleep.

Staying hydrated will help to keep the body functioning properly, and getting enough rest will help to reduce the risk of injury.

Finally, with regular exercise and physical activity, the elderly can help to limit the effects of aging on their bodies.

Using anti-aging products can also help limit the effects of aging. Anti-aging products, such as creams and serums, can help the skin to become less wrinkled and maintain youthful-looking skin.

The physical changes of aging can be difficult to cope with, both physically and emotionally. While it may seem like these changes are inevitable, there are ways to limit their effects and even overcome them in some cases. By leading a healthy lifestyle, protecting the skin from environmental factors, and using anti-aging products, you can help limit the effects of aging and keep your body looking and feeling youthful.

NUTRITION AND DIET

Nutrition and diet can play an important role in helping you stay healthy and active. Our bodies' capacity to digest and utilize nutrients declines with age. This can result in health issues like a reduced immune system, weakness, and an elevated risk of chronic diseases.

By eating a balanced diet and following nutrition principles, the elderly can improve their overall health and well-being and even slow down the effects of aging.

The Basics of Nutrition and Diet for the Elderly

Nutrition provides the body with the food and nutrients needed to sustain life and health. It is important to develop an individualized nutrition plan as you age, as your nutritional needs and abilities may differ from those of younger adults.

In general, the elderly should focus on consuming a balanced diet full of essential vitamins, minerals, and other nutrients. The diet should be high in fruits, whole grains, vegetables, healthy fats, and lean proteins while low in saturated fat, trans fat, and cholesterol.

Limiting processed foods, refined carbohydrates, and added sugars is also important.

Additionally, you should get plenty of fluids, such as water and low-fat or fat-free milk, as well as other beverages.

Eating a Balanced Diet

Consuming a well-balanced diet is essential for optimum nutrition as you age. This means eating various foods from all the food groups, including fruits, vegetables, grains, proteins, and dairy products.

The elderly should aim to include a variety of colors in their food choices, as this indicates the different nutrients present in the food.

A well-balanced diet can give you the necessary vitamins, minerals, and nutrients to stay healthy.

Fiber

Fiber helps maintain digestive health and promotes a healthy gut microbiome, which is important for overall health and longevity. It helps to regulate digestion, improve nutrient absorption, and maintain a healthy weight. It also helps reduce the risk of constipation, heart disease, and diabetes.

Fiber helps to keep blood sugar levels stable, which can help to reduce cravings for unhealthy foods.

Finally, it is also important for gut health, as it helps feed the good bacteria in the gut. Foods high in fiber, such as fruits, whole grains, and vegetables, can lower the risk of aging-related chronic diseases.

Fruits and Vegetables

Some essential components of a healthy diet for the elderly include fruits and vegetables. They are high in essential vitamins, minerals, and other nutrients and are low in calories and fat. It would help if you aimed to consume about five servings of fruits and vegetables each day in a variety of colors.

Fruits and vegetables can be eaten in various ways, including fresh, frozen, canned, or dried.

Whole Grains

Fiber and other vital nutrients are abundant in whole grains. These can help you feel satisfied for a longer period and lower your risk of developing certain illnesses, such as type 2 diabetes and heart disease.

Whole grains can be found in various foods, including whole-grain bread and pasta, oats, brown rice, quinoa, and barley.

Antioxidants

Antioxidants are compounds that protect the body from damage caused by free radicals. These free radicals are produced by various cellular processes and can cause oxidative stress, which leads to cell damage and aging. Foods rich in antioxidants, such as fruits, vegetables, nuts, and seeds, can help neutralize free radicals and prevent cellular damage.

Protein

Protein is essential for maintaining muscle mass and bone density, which tend to decrease with age. Consuming adequate amounts of protein can help slow down age-related muscle loss and maintain bone health.

An aged person's diet should include plenty of protein because it helps maintain and develop muscle. Lean proteins, such as fish, chicken, eggs, and beans, should be included in the diet. It would help if you also aimed to add a range of proteins to your diet, including plant-based proteins, such as nuts, seeds, and legumes.

Healthy Fats (Omega-3 & 6 fatty acids)

The elderly should consume healthy fats such as those in nuts, avocados, and olive oil. They give us energy as well as vital vitamins and minerals. Healthy fats can also help reduce the risk of diseases like heart disease and type 2 diabetes.

The body needs omega-3 fatty acids because it cannot create them on its own. They are essential in lowering inflammation, enhancing cognitive function, and fostering heart health. Nuts, seeds, and fatty fish all contain omega-3 fatty acids.

Limiting Unhealthy Foods

I can't overemphasize that as you grow old, you should limit or avoid foods high in saturated fat, trans fat, and cholesterol, as these can increase the risk of certain diseases. Processed foods, refined carbohydrates, and added sugars should also be limited, as they can be high in calories and low in essential vitamins and minerals. Alcohol should be consumed in moderation, as it can increase the risk of certain health issues.

Benefits of Healthy Nutrition and Diet for the Elderly

Eating a healthy diet can help the elderly maintain their overall health and well-being. It can help improve their immune system, reduce the risk of chronic diseases, and even slow down the effects of aging. Eating a balanced diet can also help you stay active, as you will have more energy and can improve your mental health and outlook on life.

Vitamin D

The immune system and bone health are both crucially dependent on vitamin D. As people age, their skin becomes less efficient at producing vitamin D, making it important to get enough from dietary sources such as fatty fish, egg yolks, and fortified foods.

In conclusion, nutrition and diet can play an important role in helping you stay healthy and active. Your overall health can be enhanced, your risk of developing chronic diseases can be decreased, and slow down the effects of aging by eating a balanced diet rich in important vitamins, minerals, and other nutrients. Eating various fruits, vegetables, whole grains, lean proteins, and healthy fats is vital to maintaining a healthy diet for the elderly.

MAINTAINING GOOD HYGIENE

Good hygiene is essential for everyone, but especially for the elderly. Not only can it help to prevent the spread of germs and illnesses, but it can also have a profound effect on the aging process. In this chapter, we'll examine the advantages and benefits of maintaining good hygiene in the elderly and how it can help to limit the effects of aging. We will also look at some practical tips for maintaining good hygiene and making it easier for you to stick to a good hygiene routine.

Benefits of Maintaining Good Hygiene in the Elderly

Maintaining proper cleanliness in the elderly has numerous psychological and physical advantages. Good hygiene can help reduce the risks of infection and illnesses, ensuring that germs and bacteria are not spread. It can also help to improve your self-esteem and confidence as you age, as looking and feeling clean can boost one's sense of worth.

Moreover, good hygiene can help to slow down the aging process. It can help keep the skin healthy and moisturized, reducing wrinkles and age spots. It can also help to reduce the risk of skin infections and other skin conditions, such as skin tags and dermatitis, which can be more common as you age.

Practical Tips for Maintaining Good Hygiene in the Elderly

You can maintain proper hygiene more easily if you follow a few simple guidelines. Firstly, ensure you have access to the right products and tools to maintain good hygiene. This includes soap, shampoo, toothbrushes, toothpaste, and other items. It's also crucial to ensure you can access these items easily, such as having them close to the bathroom or shower. Having a routine for maintaining good hygiene is also important as you age. This could include showering or bathing daily, brushing your teeth twice daily, and changing your clothes regularly.

It is also essential to make sure that the elderly person is comfortable and safe when they are carrying out their hygiene routine. This could include providing them with shower chairs, grab bars, and other products that can help to make the process easier and safer.

Finally, knowing the importance of good hygiene will go a long way, and reading books that explain the benefits and why it is important to maintain good hygiene is the way to go.

GETTING ENOUGH SLEEP

It is a well-known fact that the need for sleep decreases as we get older, but getting enough sleep is essential for everyone, regardless of your age. Your health may suffer from insomnia, and you may experience an increased risk of heart disease, stroke, depression, and even death.

Sleep deprivation can also accelerate aging and increase the risk of age-related illnesses and conditions. Fortunately, you may take measures to ensure you get enough sleep and lessen the impacts of aging on your body. This chapter will discuss the importance of getting enough sleep and how it can help limit the aging effect on you.

The Benefits of Getting Enough Sleep

Sleeping is important for overall health and well-being, especially as you age. Sleep helps the body to repair itself, and it helps to reduce stress and improve mood. It also helps to boost the immune system, improve memory and concentration, and increase energy levels.

Insomnia can have a negative impact on your health, such as an increased risk of heart disease, stroke, depression, and even death. It can also accelerate aging and increase the risk of age-related illnesses and conditions. Sleep is also important for the elderly because it helps regulate hormones and balance the body. Moreover, it helps to lessen discomfort, enhance cognitive function, and lower the chance of injury from falls.

Insomnia can lead to fatigue, confusion, and a weakened immune system. It can also increase the risk of age-related conditions such as Alzheimer's, dementia, and osteoporosis.

Tips for Getting Enough Sleep

To make sure you get adequate sleep, you can take several steps. The first step is to establish and stick to a regular sleep routine. It is easier to obtain a better night's sleep and to maintain the rhythm of your body's internal clock if you adhere to a regular bedtime and wake-up time.

It is also important to create a comfortable sleep environment. Ascertain that your bedroom is cool, quiet, and dark. Also, avoid eating, drinking, or exercising close to bedtime. These activities may keep you up at night and prevent you from sleeping properly.

Limiting your exposure to screens at least an hour before bedtime is also important. It may be difficult to fall asleep due to the blue light from displays interfering with your body's natural sleep cycle.

Finally, it is also important to avoid caffeine, alcohol, and nicotine close to bedtime. These substances can disrupt your sleep and make it challenging to achieve a restful night's sleep.

CHAPTER 3

MAINTAINING MENTAL WELLNESS

Maintaining mental wellness is one of the most important aspects to consider when aging. Mental wellness plays an important role in the overall health and well-being of the elderly, and it is important to understand how it can help them to overcome and limit the aging effect.

Mental wellness is maintaining a positive outlook and attitude toward life and the ability to think and act healthily. It can be achieved through various methods, such as exercise, healthy eating, stress management, and social activities.

As a crucial component of general health and well-being, mental wellness is significant not just for the elderly but for everyone. One of the most effective methods to preserve mental wellness is through exercise. Not only does it help to reduce stress, but it also helps to keep the body fit and strong.

Regular physical activity can help to improve mood, reduce anxiety and depression, and improve overall cognitive functioning.

Stress management is also essential for maintaining mental wellness. Stress can have a negative impact on the body and mind, and it is important to learn how to manage it effectively. Deep breathing, yoga, and other stress-reduction exercises can all assist in lowering stress levels and enhancing general well-being.

Additionally, finding ways to relax and unwind is crucial, such as spending time with friends or family, engaging in hobbies, or taking a vacation.

Let's talk about the following tips for maintaining mental wellness: (i) Keeping the brain active, (ii) Overcoming loneliness and isolation, (iii) Dealing with depression and anxiety, (iv) Staying positive and mindful, (v) Seeking professional help.

KEEPING THE BRAIN ACTIVE

As we age, our brain starts to slow down like the rest of our body. This can be disheartening for the elderly, who want to remain sharp and active. While aging brings about some cognitive decline, research has shown that the brain can be kept active, limiting the effects of aging.

In this chapter, we will explore some ways you can keep your brain active and how doing so can help them overcome and limit the effects of aging.

Benefits of Keeping the Brain Active

Keeping the brain active can help you as you age in several ways. It can help you retain your cognitive abilities and stay sharp, even as you age. It can also help prevent or delay the onset of dementia and other age-related conditions.

Additionally, engaging in activities that stimulate the brain can help you stay socially engaged and connected, which can help you remain independent for longer.

Strategies for Keeping the Brain Active

To keep your brain active, you can employ several techniques.

Maintaining social engagement is among the most crucial things. This can include participating in activities with friends and family, joining clubs or classes, and volunteering in the community.

Another way to keep the brain active is to engage in challenging activities. These can include puzzles like crosswords, jigsaw puzzles, and Sudoku.

Playing board and card games can also help keep your mind sharp. Reading books and taking classes are also great ways to engage the brain and learn new things. It is also important to stay physically active.

Aging adults can maintain their independence for longer by engaging in physical activity, which has been related to increased cognitive performance.

Additionally, physical activity can help reduce stress and improve mood, both of which can help you stay mentally sharp.

Finally, you should make sure you get enough rest. Sleep is essential to cognitive functioning, and it can help reduce stress and improve mood. Creating a regular sleep routine and getting at least seven hours of sleep per night is essential.

I have always been active, but as I have gotten older, I have become more aware of the importance of keeping my brain active. I knew I would lose it if I didn't use it, so I decided to take up activities that would help keep my brain engaged. I started reading books of all genres, trying to learn something new daily. I study books on philosophy, science, and history to broaden my perspective on the world. I also started to do puzzles, like crosswords and Sudoku, to help challenge my mind. I also took up learning new skills. I started learning how to play the guitar, knit, and spend time in the garden, challenging my brain to learn new things. I also tried helping the kids with assignments, especially painting, and drawing, which helped to stimulate my creative side.

The most important thing I did was interact with other people. Considering the nature of my job, I would have conversations with people of all ages, talking about their well-being and other topics, which really kept my brain active. I also started volunteering and helping in my local community, which made me feel good about myself and engaged my brain. All these activities have significantly improved my mental and physical health. I feel more alert and energetic than ever before and even feel like I'm aging more slowly. My mind is sharper, and I'm better able to remember things. I feel like I'm using my brain more than ever. I'm so glad I started keeping my brain active, and I would recommend it to anyone looking to improve their mental health and slow down the aging process.

Keeping the brain active is essential to stay sharp and independent for as long as possible. You can use various strategies to keep your brain active, such as staying socially engaged, engaging in activities challenging the brain, staying physically active, and getting enough rest. By using these strategies, you can limit the effects of aging on your brain and continue to enjoy life to the fullest.

OVERCOMING LONELINESS AND ISOLATION

Loneliness and isolation can be devastating for the elderly. Physical and mental changes brought on by aging can make it challenging to maintain social relationships and might result in feelings of loneliness and isolation. But there are ways to combat loneliness and isolation and help to limit the aging effects that can come with them.

Some of us are always vibrant and social at a young age. We enjoy going out with friends, attending social gatherings, and conversing with those around us. But, as we age, our ability to do these activities diminishes. Our friends may begin to drift away, and we become increasingly isolated.

Particularly, I was worried about the health of one of my aged patients, both physical and mental. I knew that loneliness and isolation could have a detrimental effect on older people, leading to depression and even physical decline. I wanted to do something to help her.

One day, I came up with an idea. I suggested to her that she join a local elder center. The center offered a variety of activities, from exercise classes to art classes and social events like dances and movie nights. It was a fantastic way for her to leave the house, meet new people, and engage in activities she enjoyed. Although she was initially hesitant, I was persistent and eventually convinced her to try out the elder center.

She was soon attending classes and social events regularly. She made new friends, and she was less isolated than before. The elder center also provided her with much-needed physical activity. As we know, exercise can help reduce the effects of aging, so it was a great way for her to stay in shape and healthy.

She and her family were so grateful that I encouraged her to join the elder center. She said it gave her a new lease on life and was her best decision in a long time. Not only did she become less isolated and depressed, but she also experienced improved physical and mental health. She was able to stay active, socialize, and enjoy life again.

I was so glad that I was able to help her overcome loneliness and isolation and that I could limit the effects of aging on her.

One of the best ways to fight loneliness and isolation is to stay connected with others. Try to stay in touch with family and friends, even if it's just an occasional phone call or letter. This can make a world of difference in your life.

I can't overemphasize the importance of maintaining physical activity, as it helps keep the body in shape and also help to combat feelings of loneliness and isolation. Participating in activities like walking, swimming, or dancing can be enjoyable and help build a sense of community and belonging.

Reading, playing games, or taking classes can help to keep the mind sharp and can help to reduce feelings of loneliness and isolation. It is also important to stay informed of current events, as this can help keep the mind sharp and provide a sense of purpose.

Staying socially active can help to limit the effects of aging. Participating in social events, such as attending plays or concerts, can help keep the mind and body engaged and provide an opportunity to build relationships with others.

Volunteering for a cause or organization can provide a sense of purpose and help build relationships with others.

Overall, loneliness and isolation can have a detrimental effect on you. But by trying to stay connected with others, stay physically active, and stay mentally and socially engaged, you can combat these feelings and limit the effects of aging. These steps allow you to lead fulfilling, meaningful lives and enjoy your golden years.

DEALING WITH DEPRESSION AND ANXIETY

Depression and anxiety can be debilitating for anyone, but they can be especially difficult to manage in the elderly. These mental health problems can negatively affect your quality of life and even speed up aging if ignored.

Fortunately, several interventions and treatments can help you manage depression and anxiety to limit the aging effect of these conditions.

The first step in managing depression and anxiety is identifying the underlying causes. You are more likely to experience depression and anxiety due to the physical and social changes that come with age, such as retirement, loss of independence, and health issues.

Additionally, you may also be more likely to experience depression and anxiety due to the increased risk of loneliness and isolation that can come with age. To effectively address the issue, it is important to comprehend the underlying factors of depression and anxiety in you. Once the potential causes of depression and anxiety in you have been identified, the next step is to create a plan to manage the condition. This plan should include both psychological and physical interventions.

Psychological therapies for depression and anxiety in the elderly can include cognitive-behavioral therapy (CBT), relaxation techniques, and problem-solving skills. You may also benefit from joining a support group or counseling sessions.

On the physical side, several interventions can be used to help manage depression and anxiety. You can release endorphins, which can assist in boosting mood and reducing stress and can help to minimize the symptoms of depression and nervousness when you perform a routine exercise. Additionally, ensuring that you are getting adequate nutrition and enough sleep and limiting the intake of caffeine and alcohol can also help to manage the symptoms of depression and anxiety.

In addition to these interventions, medication may also be necessary to manage depression and anxiety as you age. Antidepressants and anxiolytics can be effective in reducing the symptoms of depression and anxiety, but a qualified medical professional should always prescribe them. It is important to understand that while medications can be effective in managing depression and anxiety, they should not be used as a long-term solution and should instead be combined with other psychological and physical interventions. Finally, it is crucial to recognize that depression and anxiety can significantly impact your quality of life and even lead to premature aging.

As such, it is important to know the signs and symptoms of depression and anxiety to identify and address the issue quickly. With the right combination of psychological, physical, and medical interventions, depression and anxiety can be effectively managed to limit the aging effect of these conditions.

STAYING POSITIVE AND MINDFUL

The effects of aging cannot be stopped, but they can be managed and limited with the right attitude and lifestyle. Staying positive and mindful is the key to keeping the elderly healthy and happy. It is important to remember that aging is natural and that staying young at heart and in spirit is possible.

Positive thinking is an integral part of staying young. Being positive allows you to focus on life's positive aspects and appreciate what you have. It also helps you look for solutions to problems rather than dwelling on negative ones. A positive attitude can be difficult, but it is essential for good health and well-being.

Mindfulness is another important aspect of staying young. It encourages you to pay attention to your thoughts and feelings and be present. It is a way to stay in touch with your inner self and appreciate your small moments. Being mindful can help you to be aware of your own needs and to take care of yourself.

Finding elderly people activities you enjoy is crucial since it will be simpler for you to stick to a routine.

Finding a routine can provide mental stability by providing structure and predictability to daily life. Having a set of routines can help keep you organized and make managing your time and energy easier. It can also give you a sense of purpose and accomplishment. When you feel like you have a plan for your day and can stick to it, it can help you feel more in control and reduce feelings of stress and anxiety. Also, having a routine can help you stay active and engaged in your lives, which is important for maintaining a healthy mental state.

Finding activities you enjoy and making them a part of your daily routine can help you stay motivated and focused on your goals. It can also provide an opportunity for socializing and forming meaningful connections with others. All of these things can lead to improved mental well-being over time.

Staying socially connected is also important for you. Socializing with friends and family can help to reduce stress and depression, and it can also help to keep you mentally active. It is important to find activities that you enjoy, such as attending social events or joining a club.

Finally, it is crucial to stay mentally active. Mental stimulation can help to slow down the effects of aging. Learning new skills and playing brain-training games, such as crosswords and puzzles, can help to keep the mind sharp. Keeping up with current events is also crucial, as this can help reduce stress and anxiety.

SEEKING PROFESSIONAL HELP

As we age, our bodies change, and age-related illnesses and issues become increasingly common. This can be daunting and difficult, often leaving you feeling helpless and alone. Seeking professional help can be an important step in managing the effects of aging and can help to limit the impact of those effects. Professional help can come in many forms, from doctors, nurses, counselors, and psychologists. All of these types of professionals can offer support and guidance to those dealing with the effects of aging and can help limit the impact that aging has on their everyday lives.

There is a man who has been struggling with the natural effects of aging on his body. He was in constant pain, and his energy levels were so low that he could not do the things he used to enjoy. He was starting to lose hope that he would ever be able to lead a quality life again.

After living in agony for some time, he was referred to my practice. He decided to give it a try and made an appointment. When he arrived, I gave him a kind and caring welcome and listened attentively as he described his symptoms.

With my knowledge and experience, I took the time to explain the different treatments available and the potential benefits of each. I prescribed medication, physical therapy, and lifestyle changes.

Over the next few weeks, the elderly man noticed a gradual improvement in his health. He felt his energy levels increasing and his pain decreasing. He could do more of the activities he enjoyed, such as walking and gardening. The elderly man was so thankful for the professional help he received that he started telling everyone in his circle about his encounter with me.

He was so pleased with his results that he regularly visited. The elderly man was surprised to find that the effects of aging on his body had been limited and even reversed. He could now enjoy the activities he loved without worrying about pain or fatigue. He said I had truly changed his life for the better. The elderly man was so grateful for his experience that he started volunteering at a local care center. He wanted to give back and help others in the same situation he had been in.

He was proud to be a part of something that was making a difference in people's lives. The elderly man was so thankful that he had received professional help. It had made such a positive difference in his life that he was determined to continue helping others. He was a living testament to the power of professional medical care.

Medical professionals are a great resource for elderly individuals struggling with age-related illnesses. Physicians can determine any underlying medical conditions that might be speeding up the aging process and offer advice on how to alleviate symptoms.

Additionally, nurses can provide care and support to those in need, ensuring they are adequately cared for. Counselors and psychologists can also provide valuable support to elderly individuals who are struggling with the effects of aging.

Counselors can provide a safe and supportive environment to discuss aging challenges and offer strategies for coping with the physical and emotional changes associated with aging. Additionally, psychologists can provide more in-depth psychological support, helping elderly individuals work through any issues that may impact their mental health.

Besides medical and mental health professionals, other resources are available to those seeking professional help with the effects of aging. For people struggling with the effects of aging, organizations like the American Association of Retired Persons (AARP) provide a wealth of information and support. The AARP also provides programs and services that can help elderly individuals maintain their independence and offer resources for those who may need additional assistance. Finally, support groups are another great resource for elderly individuals who are struggling with the effects of aging. Support groups can provide a safe and supportive environment in which to discuss the challenges of aging and can also provide a sense of community and connection.

Seeking professional help can be a crucial step in managing the effects of aging and can help limit the impact of aging on your individual life. Medical professionals, counselors, and psychologists can provide valuable support and guidance, while organizations such as the AARP can provide resources and programs to help you maintain your independence. Additionally, support groups can provide a sense of community and connection, helping those who are struggling with the effects of aging to feel less alone.

All of these resources can be invaluable in helping you cope with the effects of aging and can help limit the impact of aging on your life.

Overall, maintaining mental wellness is an important aspect of aging gracefully and healthily. It is crucial to understand how mental wellness can be achieved through keeping the Brain Active, Overcoming Loneliness and Isolation, Dealing with Depression and Anxiety, Staying Positive and Mindful, and Seeking Professional Help. All of these aspects are essential for maintaining good mental health and well-being and can help to reduce the effects of aging. With the proper lifestyle and habits, the aging process can be made easier and more comfortable, and mental wellness can help to achieve this.

CHAPTER 4

EMBRACING EMOTIONAL CHANGES

As you age, you will often face many emotional changes. These changes can be challenging to accept, significantly impacting your quality of life. However, by embracing these emotional changes, you can learn to cope and use them to your advantage.

In this chapter, we'll look at Accepting the Loss of Loved Ones, Managing Grief and Bereavement, Dealing with Life Transitions, and Finding Purpose and Meaning. But before then, let's discuss embracing emotional changes.

One of the most common emotional changes that come with aging is a decrease in energy levels. As the body begins to break down, you often feel tired and sluggish. This can be extremely difficult to accept, as many elderly people still feel like they should be as active and energetic as they once were.

The key to overcoming this change is to embrace it. By recognizing that one's energy levels will naturally decrease as one age, you can learn to accept it and manage your energy levels to allow you to enjoy life still.

Another common emotional change that comes with aging is a decrease in motivation. As the body ages, finding the motivation to do things can become more difficult. This can be especially difficult for those who used to be very active and driven. To help overcome this, you can focus on setting small, achievable goals.

By setting achievable goals, you can find the motivation to complete them and still feel accomplished.

Aging can also lead to an increase in loneliness and isolation. People may find it more difficult to maintain relationships and find friends as they age. This can be very difficult for you to accept, as you may feel like you are being forgotten and neglected.

To mitigate these, you can join social clubs, take classes, or volunteer in their community. This can help you create meaningful relationships and feel connected to the world around you.

In the end, you can embrace emotional changes by accepting your limitations. Some hobbies that you formerly enjoyed can get harder to accomplish as the body ages. This can be difficult to accept, as it may feel like a loss of independence. To help with this, you can focus on finding activities that you can still enjoy and that are within your capabilities. This can help you still find joy and feel a sense of accomplishment.

Embracing emotional changes can be difficult, but it is an important part of coping with aging. By accepting these changes and learning to manage them, you can still find joy in life and limit the effects of aging. You can still live a whole and meaningful life with the right attitude and support.

ACCEPTING THE LOSS OF LOVED ONES

Losing a loved one is never easy for anyone, regardless of age. For the elderly, losing a partner or close family member can be especially difficult to bear.

The grief process for the elderly is often more complex than for younger people due to their greater life experiences and the fact that they are often more isolated from friends and family.

It is important to remain mindful that, while it may be difficult, it is possible to accept the loss of a loved one and use the experience to help overcome and limit the impact of aging.

The first step in accepting the loss of a loved one is to acknowledge the pain and grief you are feeling. Acknowledge this difficult time and allow yourself to feel whatever emotions arise. Allow yourself to cry, talk to friends, or spend time with family. It would help if you also took cognizant that grief is a process and that taking your time to process and heal is okay.

Once you have acknowledged your feelings, it would help to remember that moving forward with your life is okay. It is usually not easy to imagine life without your loved one, but it is important to remember that while they may be gone, the memories you share linger.

Reminiscing on the good times and remembering your loved one can be a positive and healthy way to honor their memory.

Finally, it is important to reach out for help if you need it. Many online and in-person support groups can offer a secure platform where you can express your emotions and seek guidance from others who have gone through similar experiences. If you feel overwhelmed or are struggling to cope with losing a loved one, reaching out to a professional, such as a therapist or counselor, is crucial. Accepting the loss of a loved one can be difficult and painful. However, it is possible to use the experience to help overcome and limit the effects of aging.

My mother was a strong woman, but she had her limits. She had been married to my father for over three decades, and they had been together since they were teenagers. But then, one day, my father passed away suddenly.

My mother was devastated—she had just lost the love of her life. She tried to carry on, but she felt like a piece of her had died along with him. She felt lost, confused, and alone. But she was a fighter and eventually accepted the reality of losing my father.

She learned to move on, and gradually she found a new normal. My mother was determined to keep going and make the most of her life, even without my father. She focused on what brought her joy, like spending time with children, going on walks with her friends, and gardening.

As time passed, my mother started to look and feel younger. She was able to limit the aging effect, and it made her feel a sense of renewal and hope. She was able to enjoy life again, and it was a beautiful thing to witness.

My mother was a remarkable woman, and I am so proud of her for the way she handled the loss of my father. She proved that even in the darkest times, we can still find the strength to keep going and make the most of life.

MANAGING GRIEF AND BEREAVEMENT

Grief and bereavement are common experiences of aging and can be difficult to manage. Feeling sad when a loved one passes away is not out of place, especially if we were close to them for a long time. But it can also be difficult for elderly people who may have

lost a partner or close friend and now face their own
mortality.

It is important to recognize that grief and
bereavement can have an aging effect on you and that
managing this grief can help to limit the effects of
aging.

One way to manage it is to be open about your
feelings. Don't be afraid to express your emotions to
yourself and others who can offer support. Talking to
someone who may have experienced a similar loss can
be helpful, as they can provide insight and
understanding.

Grief and bereavement can be managed by engaging
in things dear and pleasurable to you. These activities
include socializing with friends and family, joining
groups, or engaging in hobbies and interests.

Participating in activities can help to provide a sense
of purpose and routine, which can help to ease the
pain of grief and bereavement. Additionally, activities
can help create a sense of belonging, giving elderly
people a sense of comfort.

Exercising is another activity that can help to manage grief and bereavement in the elderly. Exercise can help reduce stress levels and improve physical and mental health. It can be done at home or in a group setting and tailored to the individual's needs and abilities.

Spending time outdoors can also be beneficial for managing grief and bereavement. Admiring nature's beauty can help ease tension and promote a sense of tranquility and peace.

It can help to provide a sense of connectivity to the world around us. This can help counter the sense of isolation that can come with aging and provide a feeling of belonging.

Engaging in spiritual activities can also help manage grief and bereavement. Spiritual activities can include praying, meditating, or engaging in worship. These activities can provide a sense of peace and can help to provide comfort and support.

Engaging in spiritual activities can help to provide a sense of connection to something larger than oneself, which can help to provide a sense of security and acceptance.

Finally, it is important to remember that grief and bereavement are natural and normal experiences of aging. The reality that there's no "right" or "wrong" method of handling these emotions must be understood. What is important is to find activities and coping strategies that work for you and allow you to move through the grieving process healthily. By engaging in activities that can help to manage grief and bereavement, and by finding support from those around you, you can help to limit the aging effect on yourself.

DEALING WITH LIFE TRANSITION

Irrespective of age, life transitions can be particularly difficult. People's social and economic circumstances, as well as their physical and mental health, may change as they get older. Although these changes can cause stress and anxiety for the elderly, there are ways to help them manage and cope with transitions.

Certain life transitions can mitigate the impacts of aging on you, and this chapter will offer tips on how to help you adjust to and cope with these changes. When we reach our elderly years, our bodies and minds are no longer as agile as they once were. We might discover that our stamina and mental acuity have diminished. We may also experience changes in our social and economic situation.

As we age, we may face the challenges of living on a fixed income, changes in relationships, and even the transition to a retirement home. These changes can create a great deal of stress and anxiety for the elderly.

However, life transitions can also be a source of strength for you. Through these changes, you can gain control over your lives and find new ways to live life to the fullest. With the help of family and friends, you can learn to manage and cope with transitions.

One way to manage life transitions is to develop a plan. Before making any changes, it is important to take the time to consider all the factors involved. This includes making decisions about finances, housing, and medical care. It is also essential to consider the emotional and psychological implications of the changes. You can reduce stress and anxiety by dedicating yourself to planning and preparedness.

Another way to help the elderly cope with life transitions is to provide emotional support. This can be done through conversation, listening, and understanding. It is important to be patient and understanding and to allow the elderly to express their feelings without judgment. By providing emotional support, the elderly can feel more secure and accepted and be more able to cope with the changes.

A particular patient in his eighties had recently been admitted to my hospital. He had difficulty managing his emotions, and his family was concerned about his well-being. As his doctor, I knew he needed to feel heard and understood. I began by having a conversation with him about his life, his experiences, and his worries. I made sure to listen carefully, without judgment or interruption.

I could see that he struggled with his age and the physical changes it brought. I empathized with his feelings and told him it was okay to express his emotions. Initially, he was hesitant, but eventually, he opened up.

He revealed the pain and fear hidden beneath the surface as he shared his story. He told me about his sadness at seeing his friends and family members pass away and regret that he could not do more for them. I provided a safe space for him to express his feelings. I listened attentively and asked questions to help him better understand and process his emotions. I assured him he wasn't overacting for feeling the way he did and that his emotions were legitimate. I also let him know that he was not alone in his struggles.

Through our conversations, the octogenarian was able to recognize his emotions and begin to cope with them. His family noticed a difference in his mood and behavior.

He eventually made a full recovery and was able to enjoy the rest of his life with his loved ones. I'm glad I could help him by providing the emotional support he needed, and I am particularly joyous that I was able to make a difference in his life.

Another way to help the elderly cope with life transitions is to provide them with opportunities for meaningful activities. This can include activities such as volunteer work, gardening, or socializing. These activities can help to keep you physically active and mentally engaged. They can also provide an outlet to express emotions and feelings.

Finally, it is important to recognize the importance of maintaining a healthy lifestyle. Our body's capacity for some tasks decreases as we become older. Modifying activities to reduce the risk of injury or illness is important. Eating a healthy diet, regular exercise, and adequate rest can help you maintain your physical and mental health. By helping the elderly manage and cope with life transitions, we can help them to overcome and limit the effects of aging on their lives. Through planning and preparation, emotional support, meaningful activities, and a healthy lifestyle, you can live life to the fullest and enjoy your golden years.

FINDING PURPOSE AND MEANING

The sense of being disconnected from the world around one's self grows as one ages. With physical changes, you can feel increasingly isolated and feel like you are just waiting for the end of your life.

However, finding life's purpose and meaning can help overcome these feelings.

The first step to finding purpose and meaning is identifying what is important to you. What are your values, goals, and passions? What makes you feel alive and excited? What do you want to accomplish or experience? Taking the time to reflect on these questions can help you to find a sense of purpose and meaning. Once you know what is important to you, it's time to start working towards that purpose and meaning. This could be anything from taking up a new hobby to volunteering in your community.

There are countless ways to make a difference in the world and to do something meaningful. Even if it's something small, like spending time with a grandchild, it can make a huge difference in the life of the elderly.

In addition to finding purpose and meaning, it's also important for you to focus on staying active and healthy. Exercise can help improve physical and mental health and can be a great way to stay connected with the world around you.

Finding activities you enjoy and ensuring you're doing them regularly is important. Socializing is another important factor in staying healthy as you age. Staying connected with family, friends, and the community is important.

Whether it's attending religious gatherings, joining a club, or simply going out for coffee with a friend, staying socially connected can help you to feel less isolated.

Finally, it's important to maintain a positive attitude and outlook. Negative thoughts can be damaging, so focusing on the good things in life is important. Always try to find the good in everything and be grateful for what you have.

With the right attitude and outlook, you can continue to find joy and purpose in life despite the physical changes that come with aging.

CHAPTER 5

THE SHRINKING SOCIAL CIRCLE

As you age, your social circles tend to shrink, and this can become a problem, as social interaction is essential for the elderly. Social interaction can help keep the mind active and even help reduce the effects of aging on you.

In this chapter, we will explore how a shrinking social circle can be reversed and how it can help to limit the effects of aging on the elderly. First, it is important to understand why a shrinking social circle is a problem for the elderly.

As people age, their physical and mental capabilities inevitably decline. At the same time, their social circle tends to shrink, as it is more difficult for them to meet new people and maintain relationships with existing friends and family. This might bring about feelings of isolation and loneliness, which can harm one's physical and mental health.

Several measures can be taken to counter the effects of a shrinking social circle. One of the most effective is to create opportunities for the elderly to interact with other people. This can be performed in many ways by joining an elder center or volunteer organization or simply spending time with other elderly people in the community. This can help create a sense of community and provide a social outlet for the elderly.

Another way to help limit the effects of aging on the elderly is to encourage them to stay active. Age-related physical symptoms, including joint stiffness and impaired balance, can be lessened with regular exercise.

Additionally, physical activity can help to improve mental health, as it can help to reduce stress and depression. Encouraging the elderly to participate in physical activities can also be a wonderful approach to keeping them socially active.

Finally, it is important to make sure that the elderly are getting the necessary nutrition and adequate rest. Poor nutrition and lack of sleep can contribute to the physical effects of aging and lead to mental fatigue and depression.

Age-related changes in aged people can be slowed down by eating a nutritious diet and obtaining adequate rest.

STAYING CONNECTED WITH FAMILY AND FRIENDS

Irrespective of age, staying connected to family and friends can be a powerful way to help overcome several challenges and limit the aging effects of time for the aged. Aging is often said to be inevitable, but staying socially connected to those we care about can make a huge difference in our emotional and physical well-being. Although aging is a natural process, older people may find it particularly challenging to adjust to the changes that come with it. From physical changes to cognitive decline, the aging process can be both challenging and isolating.

It is important for family and friends of elderly individuals to stay connected with them, recognizing the importance of regular contact, emotional support, and understanding. Being social has a multitude of benefits for elderly individuals, especially for those who are living alone. Staying socially connected can help to ease feelings of loneliness, depression, and anxiety while providing a sense of companionship and community.

It can also help to keep the mind active, reduce stress levels, and even help to maintain physical health. Family and friends can help you stay connected through regular visits or phone calls. This can be an invaluable source of emotional support and companionship, helping to keep you feeling connected and valued.

If a friend or family member is unable to visit regularly, there are other ways to stay connected, such as sending letters, emails, or text messages. Another great way for elderly individuals to stay connected is through technology. Many elders use social media such as Facebook and Skype to stay connected with family and friends. This can be a great way to share stories, photos, and updates.

Additionally, many websites and apps are specifically designed to help elderly individuals stay connected with their loved ones. With these platforms, you may be able to communicate with distant relatives and keep tabs on loved ones' daily activities.

Staying socially connected can also help elderly individuals to maintain their physical health. Research has shown that socially connected individuals have better overall physical and mental health. They have a lower risk of experiencing mental health issues such as depressive disorders, anxiety, and others. They also have lower blood pressure and are likelier to maintain a healthy lifestyle.

Staying connected with family and friends can also help to limit the effects of aging. It can help keep your mind sharp and alert while providing a sense of purpose and meaning. By staying connected to your loved ones, you remain engaged and active, which can help to slow down the aging process.

In conclusion, staying connected with family and friends is an important way to help elderly individuals to overcome and limit the aging effects of time. Regular contact, companionship, and emotional support can make a huge difference in the physical and mental well-being of elderly individuals. Technology can also provide a great way for elderly individuals to stay connected with their loved ones, even if they are living far away. By staying connected, elderly individuals can keep their minds sharp, reduce stress levels, and even help to maintain physical health.

The following are some strategies I employ to maintain contact with patients:

1. I use social media platforms like Twitter, Facebook, and Instagram to stay in touch with them. I share updates on medical news and treatments and any new developments in my practice as related to their well-being. I also use these platforms to answer questions or advise patients.
2. Email is also a great way I use to stay connected with patients, especially when I want to send out reminders or updates about their appointments or treatments. I also use email to answer any questions or provide advice for patients.
3. I invite patients to join online patient communities to connect with other patients. This is effective as it helps increase patient

engagement and satisfaction. It allows patients to share their experiences and learn from one another, which can be beneficial to all parties.

4. I offer telemedicine visits to provide convenient care to patients who cannot make it into the office. Through telemedicine, patients connect with me from the comfort of their own homes without having to leave the house or take time off from work. It also eliminates wait times, travel, and parking expenses and helps patients save time and money.

By staying connected with the aged through social platforms, email, and video calls, you can foster better relationships and ensure they get the care they need. Properly caring for the aged can help you establish a rapport with them and gain their trust.

BUILDING NEW RELATIONSHIPS

Building new relationships can be a great way for the elderly to combat the effects of aging. As people age, they may experience several physical ailments and changes that can limit their ability to interact with others. In addition, they may experience loneliness, isolation, and a lack of emotional support. Building new relationships can help to combat these negative effects of aging.

The first step in building new relationships is to recognize the need for them. This can be difficult for you as you age, as you may feel you have already made all the friends you need or that it is too late to start making new ones. It is important to understand that relationships are an important part of life and that building new ones can be a great way for you to stay connected and engaged with the world.

The next action is to look for approaches to meeting new people. This can be done in several ways. For example, joining a local elders' social club or attending community events can be great ways to meet new people.

Volunteering is another terrific way to connect with others. It can help to make a difference in the community, and it can also be a great way to meet new people. Once a person has found ways to meet new people, taking the initiative to get to know them is important. This can include inviting them out for coffee, a walk, or dinner. It is also important to be open and friendly, as this will help to create a foundation for a strong relationship.

When it comes to building relationships with people as you age, it is important to remember that communication is key. It is important to listen to their stories and experiences and to ask questions. This will help to create a strong foundation of understanding between you and them.

Finally, it is important to show appreciation and gratitude. Showing appreciation and gratitude can help create a connection and trust. Showing appreciation and gratitude is also a great way to make people feel valued and respected.

Aside from building new relationships with other people, you also need to build new relationships with your body. I've been building a new relationship with my body for the past few years. This has been the best decision I've ever made. I used to think that aging was inevitable and that I had to accept and live with it. I thought that my body would deteriorate as I got older and that I would have to live with the physical and mental effects of aging. But that's not the case. I've come to understand that aging can be managed and limited.

I'm learning to treat my body with respect and understanding and to nourish it with healthy food and exercise. I'm also taking steps to ensure I get enough sleep and manage my stress levels. I'm reclaiming control over my physical and mental health by building this new relationship with my body.

I'm learning to appreciate the small changes that come with age, like wrinkles and grey hair. I'm also learning to focus on the things I can still do and enjoy, like spending time with my family and doing the things I love. The results have been incredible.

I'm feeling energized and healthier than ever before. I'm no longer afraid of aging and embracing the changes that come with it. I'm confident that, by building this new relationship with my body, I'll enjoy a healthy and happy life well into my later years.

You can also build a new relationship with your body by doing the following:

1. **Understand the changes you're going through:** Aging is a natural process, and it's

important to understand your body's changes.
Educate yourself on the physical and emotional
changes that can come with aging and how those
changes may affect your relationship with your body.

2. **Respect your body's limits:** As we age, our
bodies can no longer do what they once did.
Recognize that your body has changed and respect its
limits. Do not push yourself to do something that
could cause harm.

3. **Practice self-compassion:** Being kind to
yourself is essential for building a healthy relationship
with your body. Don't focus on what you can't do;
appreciate what your body can do.

4. **Focus on wellness rather than appearance:**
As we age, we should shift from physical appearance
to overall well-being. Take steps to stay physically and
mentally active, and nourish your body with healthy
food.

5. **Celebrate your body:** Celebrate your body's
accomplishments, no matter how small. Please focus
on the things your body can do and be proud of all it
has achieved.

6. **Surround yourself with positivity:** Being around uplifting individuals might help you feel better about your body and improve your self-esteem. Spend time with those that help you feel positive about your body and self-worth.

7. **Reach out for support:** Building a new relationship with your body can be hard, so don't hesitate to reach out for support. Talk to friends and family, or seek help from a professional if needed.

STRENGTHENING ROMANTIC RELATIONSHIP

Aging is something that we all must go through. It is a natural part of life and cannot be avoided. As I grew older, I was constantly reminded of this reality. I had watched my mother grow old and often had first-hand information about health issues that came with age. It was easy to become discouraged and feel that my life would become more difficult as I aged. However, I found a source of strength and comfort in my strong romantic relationship.

I had been with my partner for many years, and I could tell that our connection was deep and meaningful. We shared experiences, communicated openly, and worked through difficult times together. This made us closer and gave me a sense of security. I knew that no matter what happened, I could rely on my partner to be there.

The strength of our relationship also had a positive effect on my physical health. As we aged, my partner and I still found ways to stay active and connected. We would go for walks, participate in activities, and spend time with each other. This kept us both physically and mentally healthy. We also made sure to take time for ourselves and to take care of our individual needs.

My partner and I also had a solid emotional connection. We could talk about our feelings and share our thoughts and experiences. This allowed us to stay in touch with each other and to support each other through various stages of life. We were able to be honest, and open with each other, which made our relationship even stronger. Our strong connection also helped me to limit the effects of aging. Every day, I was reminded of how much my partner cared for me and how much they were willing to do for me. This made me feel less alone and gave me the strength to push through difficult times. I could stay positive and find joy in the moments we shared.

My strong romantic relationship was a source of comfort and strength throughout my life. It enabled me to stay physically and mentally healthy, and it helped me to limit the effects of aging. I was reminded of how much my partner cared for me, and our connection gave me the courage to face the challenges of aging. Our relationship was a source of security and love I could always rely on.

Age-related physical, mental, and emotional changes can make living a healthy and satisfying life challenging. Fortunately, strengthening a romantic relationship can help you overcome and limit the aging effects. Older people often experience physical changes that can decrease mobility, strength, and energy. This can make it challenging to take part in activities they used to enjoy, such as going on walks or going out with friends.

Strengthening a romantic relationship can help you stay active and engaged. Having a partner to go on walks with or to join you on outings can provide the motivation and support you need to remain physically active.

Additionally, a romantic partner can provide emotional and psychological support to help you cope with the physical changes associated with aging.

Mental changes are also common in the elderly. Cognitive decline, memory loss, and difficulty focusing affect their ability to think clearly and remember vital information. Strengthening a romantic relationship can help you stay mentally active and engaged. Having someone to talk to, reminisce with, and share memories with can provide the mental stimulation and emotional support you need to maintain a healthy and active mind.

A partner can help you stay organized and on top of your day-to-day tasks and activities, which can help you maintain your mental clarity. Finally, the elderly may experience emotional changes like loneliness, depression, and anxiety. These feelings can be difficult to cope with, especially as you age. Strengthening a romantic relationship can allow you to express your feelings and share your thoughts with someone you trust. Having a partner to talk to can also help you stay connected to the world around you and provides you with a sense of purpose and belonging.

BUILDING A NEW SUPPORT SYSTEM

I had been considering for a long the notion of building a new support system to aid me in limiting the impacts of aging. My retirement age from a career that had been both rewarding and challenging draws closer, and I knew that I had to find a way to keep myself active and engaged in life. I have enough information on various aging management techniques, such as maintaining an active lifestyle, eating healthy food, and enjoying enough rest and sleep. But I wanted to take things a step further and build a system that would actively help me counter the physical and cognitive effects of aging.

I began by looking at the research and literature on aging. My research reveals that physical activity is important for maintaining physical and cognitive health in later life. Regular exercise can help maintain muscle strength, reduce the risk of falls, improve cardiovascular health, and maintain a healthy weight. Proper nutrition is also essential for helping to limit the effects of aging. Foods high in nutrients, like fruits, vegetables, whole grains, protein, and healthy fats, can help reduce inflammation, fight disease, and maintain cognitive health. Social engagement is also important for helping to reduce the effects of aging as it helps to reduce loneliness, promote social connections, and provide mental stimulation.

On the other hand, stress, depression, and inadequate rest can exacerbate the effects of aging. Stress can cause increased levels of cortisol, which is linked to accelerated aging. Depression can cause a lack of motivation and energy, leading to an inactive lifestyle and unhealthy eating habits. Inadequate rest can lead to fatigue, which can cause decreased levels of physical activity and poor nutrition. All of these factors can lead to accelerated aging. Armed with this knowledge, I set out to create a plan for myself.

First, I committed to staying physically active.

I decided to start with walking because it is an activity that is easy to do, can be done indoors or outdoors, and doesn't require any special equipment. I also challenged myself by walking in places like parks, trails, and hills. I incorporated some light weights into my workouts and began doing yoga, which is great for flexibility and balance.

Second, I made sure to eat a balanced diet. I focused my meals on fresh fruits and vegetables, lean proteins, and complex carbohydrates. I tried to limit my intake of processed foods and sugar, as well as alcohol and caffeine. I also made sure to drink plenty of water throughout the day.

Third, I made sure to get enough rest and sleep. I used a sleep tracker to ensure I slept well each night. I also got up early enough for quality rest before starting my day.

Finally, I focused on staying socially engaged. I joined a local elder center, where I could meet with other aged people and participate in activities. I also started volunteering to help with activities for the elderly.

Additionally, I made sure to stay in touch with friends and family, and I even started a blog to keep my mind active and engaged. Combining physical activity, proper nutrition, adequate rest, and social engagement has benefited me.

I have noticed a marked improvement in my physical health, as well as my mental and emotional well-being, such as decreased energy levels, weaker muscles, and decreased cognitive function.

By building a new support system and taking proactive steps to limit the effects of aging, I have been able to stay healthy and active well into my old age. I have also enjoyed life more as I have maintained my physical and mental health. I believe that this proactive approach to aging has been key to my success in managing the effects of aging and maintaining a healthy lifestyle.

Let me share with you the strategies for building a comprehensive and efficient support system that will help the elderly overcome and limit the effects of aging.

Step 1: Assessing the Needs of the Elderly

The first step in building a new support system for the elderly is to assess their needs. This assessment should include physical and mental health and social and emotional needs. It should also include an evaluation of their living situation and other factors contributing to the aging process. This assessment can be done through interviews, questionnaires, and observation.

Step 2: Creating a Plan of Action

Once the needs of the elderly have been assessed, the next step is to create a plan of action. This strategy needs to have clear objectives and targets that will aid in overcoming and reducing the impacts of aging on them. The plan should also include strategies for achieving these goals and objectives, such as providing access to resources and services, providing education and support, and creating a support network.

Step 3: Finding the Right Resources

Once the plan of action has been created, the next step is to identify the resources that will be necessary to implement the plan. This may include physical resources such as medical care, legal assistance, housing, and transportation. It may also include social resources such as support groups and community organizations. This step may also involve finding financial resources, such as grants, scholarships, or loans.

Step 4: Implementing the Plan

Once the necessary resources have been identified, the next step is implementing the plan. This may involve providing direct assistance to the elderly, such as helping them apply for resources and services or educating them about aging and its effects. It may also involve creating a support network, such as a support group or a mentoring program.

Step 5: Providing Ongoing Support

The final step in building a new support system for the elderly is to provide ongoing support. This may involve regular check-ins to ensure the elderly are doing well, offering advice and assistance when needed, and providing emotional and social support. It might also entail standing up for the elderly and satisfying their needs.

Building a new support system for the elderly to help them overcome and limit the effects of aging is a challenging but rewarding process.

CHAPTER 6

UNDERSTANDING AND OVERCOMING AGEISM

Ageism is an issue that affects people of all ages but is especially difficult for elderly individuals. Ageism is "prejudice or discrimination against a person or group based on age."

It is often expressed through jokes, stereotypes, and negative attitudes. Ageism can lead to feelings of isolation and loneliness and affect physical and mental health. Comprehending ageism's underlying roots and the most effective ways to combat them is critical.

The most common ageist attitudes come from beliefs about what it means to be "old," such as the idea that older people cannot do the same activities as younger people. These beliefs can create barriers for older people, who may find it difficult to find jobs, access services, or even interact with others.

The first step in overcoming ageism is to recognize it when it arises. It is important to know how ageism manifests in language and attitudes and to speak up when it is encountered. It is also important to remember that there is no single definition of "old" and that age is just a number.

The second step is to challenge ageist attitudes and stereotypes. Speak up if you hear someone making an ageist joke or comment or see someone treating an older person differently. It is important to remember that age is not an indicator of ability or worth and that everyone deserves respect regardless of age.

The third step is to take real action towards creating a more age-inclusive society. This includes advocating for policies that support older individuals, such as increasing access to healthcare and services for elderly people. It also includes connecting with and supporting community organizations that support older individuals.

Finally, it is important to recognize that ageism is a complex issue and that overcoming it requires a multi-faceted approach. It is essential to focus on changing attitudes and behaviors and creating an environment that is more supportive of older individuals.

This includes creating opportunities for older people to participate in activities and engage in meaningful connections.

By understanding and overcoming ageism, we can help limit the aging effect on the elderly and ensure everyone is treated with respect and dignity.

RECOGNIZING THE EFFECTS OF AGEISM

Recognizing the effects of ageism is an important step in helping to overcome and limit the aging effect on the elderly. By recognizing the signs of ageism, it is possible to take action to help protect the rights and welfare of elderly individuals. When recognizing the effects of ageism, it is crucial to recognize the signs that ageism may be present. Some of the most common signs of ageism include:

- **Prejudice or stereotyping of elderly people**: This is a sign of ageism because it treats elderly people differently or unfairly based on age. This can include assuming that older people are slow, weak, or unable to do certain things. It implies that elderly people cannot participate in activities or contribute to society like younger people, which is untrue. Ageism can lead to discrimination, which can seriously affect elderly people.

- **Treating elderly people as if they are invisible or unimportant**: This is a sign of ageism. It reflects a negative attitude and stereotype toward elderly people, assuming they are unimportant enough to be seen or heard. The elderly may experience feelings of isolation and loneliness due to this treatment, which is unethical and disrespectful.

- **Treating elderly people with less respect than other age groups**: Treating elderly people with less respect than other age groups is a sign of ageism because it implies that elderly people are not worthy of the same level of respect as other age groups. It also means that elderly people have less value than other age groups, which is a form of discrimination.

- **Excluding elderly people from activities or services**: Excluding elderly people from activities or services is a sign of ageism because it denies people of a certain age group access to opportunities or resources that are available to other age groups. This type of discrimination can limit the elderly from participating in activities that could benefit their physical and mental health, as well as their overall well-being. Ageism can also result in feelings of marginalization and isolation, which can be detrimental to an aged person's quality of life and self-esteem.

- **Refusing to hire or promote elderly people:** Refusing to hire or promote elderly people is a sign of ageism because it is discrimination based on a person's age. It can be assumed that the reason for not hiring or promoting elderly people is because of their age rather than their qualifications, which is a form of ageism. This type of ageism is commonly seen in the workplace and can be a form of employment discrimination.

- **Making assumptions about elderly people based on their age**: Ageism is discrimination based on an individual's age, and it manifests itself when assumptions are made about elderly individuals based only on their age. It can include making assumptions or stereotypes about an individual's abilities, interests, or behaviors based solely on their age rather than their experience or characteristics. Ageism can lead to the exclusion of older people from certain opportunities or the denial of rights and privileges available to people of other ages.

- **Excluding elderly people from decision-making processes**: Excluding elderly people from decision-making processes is a sign of ageism because it implies that elderly people are incapable of participating in decision-making processes and are thus not worthy of having a say in those processes. This type of exclusion is a form of discrimination based on age. It denies the elderly the opportunity to contribute their wisdom, knowledge, and experience to decision-making.

- **Denying elderly people access to services or resources**: Denying elderly people access to services or resources is a sign of ageism because it discriminates against them based solely on their age. This type of discrimination is unjust and can lead to negative health outcomes for elderly people and restricted access to necessary resources. It is also a form of inequality that can lead to social exclusion and alienation.

- **Discriminating against elderly people in terms of housing, employment, or health care:** Discriminating against elderly people in terms of housing, employment, or health care is a sign of ageism because it is a form of prejudice and stereotyping based on someone's age. Ageism is the discrimination of people based on age and can manifest itself in different ways, such as limiting the elderly's access to certain jobs, housing, or health care. Denying elderly people the same opportunities as other age groups is a form of discrimination that reinforces negative stereotypes and the idea that elderly people are not as capable or useful as younger people.

- **Treating elderly people differently based on their age**: Treating elderly people differently based on their age is a sign of ageism because it implies that elderly people should be judged or treated differently solely because of their age. This form of discrimination is discriminatory and is an example of ageism. It assumes that all elderly people are the same and that the same rules should not apply to them as to other age groups. This ageism reinforces stereotypes and is an unfair way to treat people.

- **Discriminating against elderly people in terms of education or social activities**: Discriminating against elderly people in terms of education or social activities is a sign of ageism because it is an act of prejudice or discrimination based on a person's age. It implies that elderly people cannot learn or participate in activities, which is not true. Ageism also denies elderly people the respect and opportunities that they deserve.

It is important to take action when it comes to overcoming and limiting the effects of ageism. Several steps can be taken to fight ageism and help protect the rights and welfare of elderly individuals.

First, it is important to recognize and challenge ageism when it occurs. Should you witness or experience ageism, speaking out and challenging the behavior is important. This can be done in various ways, such as talking to the person responsible for the ageism, making a complaint to an authority, or taking legal action.

Second, it is important to raise awareness about ageism and the issues that elderly people face. Raising awareness can help to reduce the stigma associated with aging and can help to create a more inclusive and understanding society. This can be done through education, media campaigns, and other initiatives.

Third, it is important to support policies and initiatives that protect the rights and welfare of elderly people. This can include advocating for policies that protect the rights of elderly people in terms of housing, employment, healthcare, education, and other areas.

Finally, it is important to support and value elderly people in our communities. By doing so, we can help to create a more inclusive and supportive environment for elderly people and help to limit the effects of ageism.

By recognizing the effects of ageism and taking action to fight it, it is possible to help overcome and limit the aging effect on the elderly. By speaking out, raising awareness, and supporting policies and initiatives that protect the rights and welfare of elderly people, we can work together to create a more inclusive and understanding society.

CHALLENGING STEREOTYPES AND PREJUDICES

We all face prejudice and stereotypes in our lives. It can be based on age, gender, race, and sexual orientation, among other things. Challenging these stereotypes and prejudices can be difficult, especially regarding the elderly. It can be hard to avoid the "ageism" in our society or the feeling that older people are not valued as much as younger people. But overcoming these stereotypes and prejudices is possible and can help limit the aging effect on the elderly.

Stereotypes and prejudices are a form of discrimination. They involve making assumptions about people based on appearance, beliefs, or behavior. Stereotypes are based on generalizations and can be negative or positive. Prejudices are based on negative assumptions and can have damaging effects on people.

Both can lead to ageism. Ageism is the belief that older people are less valuable or not as capable as younger people. This can lead to discrimination in the workplace, housing, and health care. The elderly may experience emotions of isolation and loneliness as a result.

The first step in challenging stereotypes and prejudices is to understand them. We must be conscious of the prejudices and preconceptions that exist in our society and how they may affect the elderly. We also need to recognize our biases and prejudices and how they can affect how we interact with older people.

Once we know our biases and prejudices, we can start to challenge them. We can start by being open to conversations about ageism and by listening to the experiences of older people. We can also challenge ageist assumptions and language when we hear them. We can also help to reduce the aging effect on the elderly by engaging in activities that help to reduce loneliness and isolation.

This can include volunteering in local elder centers, participating in intergenerational activities, or even trying to stay in touch with elderly family members and friends.

Challenging stereotypes and prejudices can help to limit the aging effect on the elderly. It can help to reduce discrimination and feelings of loneliness and isolation. We can all take steps to challenge our own biases and prejudices and to be open to conversations about ageism. We can also help to reduce the aging effect on the elderly by engaging in activities that help to reduce loneliness and isolation.

ADVOCATING FOR OLDER ADULTS

Advocating for older adults is an important part of supporting them as they age. It is a way for them to ensure that their needs are being met, that their rights are being respected, and that their voices are heard. When we advocate for older adults, we are speaking out on behalf of those who may not have the confidence or ability to do so themselves. We are helping to ensure that the elderly are not marginalized or treated unfairly.

We are also helping to ensure that their needs and wishes are taken into account in the decision-making process.

It also helps to limit the effect of aging on them. As people age, they may become more vulnerable to neglect and abuse, and they may not have the ability to speak up for themselves. By advocating for them, we can help to ensure that they are being treated with respect and dignity and that their rights are being protected.

Advocacy for older adults can take many different forms. It can involve speaking up on their behalf in social settings, such as at their doctor's office or in their community.

It can involve writing letters to government officials or organizations to express their concerns. It can also involve attending meetings and speaking on their behalf to ensure that their views are being heard.

It can also involve advocating on their behalf in the legal arena. This may include filing a complaint or grievance if they have been mistreated or their rights have been violated. It may also include providing support and assistance to them throughout the legal process to ensure that their rights are being protected.

It also involves educating them about their rights and helping them understand how to access the resources and services that are available to them. This can include helping them understand the importance of having an adequate retirement income, understanding what their insurance covers, and knowing how to access home health care services.

Advocating for older adults can help ensure that their voices are heard and that they receive the best possible care. It can also help limit the effects of aging on them by ensuring that their rights are respected and that they are receiving the services they need. By speaking out for them, we can ensure that people live as comfortably as possible as they age.

PROMOTING AGE-INCLUSIVE POLICIES

Age-inclusive policies are an important aspect of promoting the well-being of the aged. It ensures that everyone can access the same services and opportunities available to the general population regardless of age.

These policies benefit the elderly, giving them the same rights and benefits available to all individuals, regardless of age. The first step in promoting age-inclusive policies is to ensure that age is not a factor when providing services and opportunities. Age shouldn't be a factor in determining who qualifies for a specific program or service; instead, each person should be considered on their own merits. This helps to ensure that the elderly are not discriminated against simply because of their age and that they have access to the same services and opportunities as other individuals.

Another critical aspect of promoting age-inclusive policies is ensuring the elderly are included in decision-making processes. This means that their voices should be heard and their opinions respected when decisions about services, policies, and programs affect their well-being. It also means their needs and preferences should be considered when designing and implementing services and policies.

Age-inclusive policies should also be implemented to ensure that the elderly can remain active and engaged in the community. This means providing the elderly with access to transportation, housing, and other amenities that make it easier for them to remain independent and active. It also means providing opportunities for them to participate in activities that promote their health and well-being, such as exercise and social activities.

Finally, age-inclusive policies should ensure that the elderly have access to the same healthcare services and treatments as the rest of the population. This means providing access to necessary medical treatments and services, regardless of age, so the elderly can receive the necessary care to stay healthy and active.

Overall, promoting age-inclusive policies is important in ensuring that the elderly population can access the same services, opportunities, and healthcare as everyone else. By doing so, we can help to limit the impact of aging on the elderly and ensure that they can remain healthy and active in their communities.

CELEBRATING DIVERSITY AND INCLUSIVITY

Diversity and inclusivity are essential elements of successful aging; celebrating them helps to create a vibrant and supportive community enriched by its members' varied backgrounds, experiences, and perspectives. In this way, you can benefit from the support of a diverse and inclusive network of friends and family members, building strong relationships and limiting the aging effect on you.

To celebrate diversity and inclusivity, it is important to recognize and appreciate the different backgrounds, values, and experiences of people in the community. This can be done through educational initiatives, such as events, seminars, or workshops focusing on understanding different cultures, histories, and religions.

Also, by recognizing and celebrating the unique experiences of individuals from different cultures, elders can gain insight into their own life stories and values, building a stronger sense of self and self-esteem. In addition to understanding and appreciating different cultures, celebrating diversity and inclusivity is also important to help reduce loneliness and isolation in the elderly.

By creating a community of people from different backgrounds, elders can form meaningful relationships, providing them with emotional support and companionship. In this way, elders can find comfort and joy in the company of different people, reducing the feeling of loneliness and helping to limit the aging effect on them. It is also important to remember that celebrating diversity and inclusivity is not just about understanding different cultures and backgrounds. It is also about creating an atmosphere of acceptance and respect for all individuals, regardless of their age, race, gender, sexual orientation, or any other characteristic. This can be done through activities and events that foster an environment of understanding and acceptance, such as intergenerational programs designed to unite people of all ages and backgrounds.

Ultimately, celebrating diversity and inclusivity can help to limit the aging effect on the elderly. By creating a supportive and inclusive community that recognizes and respects its members' varied backgrounds, experiences, and perspectives, elders can benefit from strong relationships and greater emotional support, reducing loneliness and isolation and helping promote healthy aging.

CHAPTER 7

PLANNING FOR THE FUTURE

As we age, we often feel like our lives is slipping away. We may feel like we don't have much control over our future and that our age limits us from doing the things we used to enjoy. But planning for the future can help reduce the aging effect and ensure we make the most of our later years.

The first step in planning for the future is to set realistic goals. This means looking at your current situation and creating achievable goals for the future. Start by making small, attainable goals, like taking a course or learning a new skill. As you progress, you can increase the difficulty of your goals and challenge yourself further.

Another important step in planning for the future is to create a budget. This will help you manage your finances and ensure that you can cover all of your expenses.

When creating a budget, it is important to factor in any medical or insurance costs and any additional costs you may incur due to your age.

Finally, it is important to stay physically and mentally active. Exercise and physical activity can help to reduce the aging effect by keeping your body strong and healthy.

Also, engaging in mental activities, such as reading or playing games, can help to keep your mind sharp. Following these steps can help reduce the aging effect and ensure you make the most of your later years.

Planning for the future can also help to provide a sense of purpose and direction, which can help to make your life more meaningful. So start planning today and make the most of your golden years.

CREATING AN ESTATE PLAN

Drafting an estate plan is one of the most crucial steps in future planning. A series of legal documents known as an estate plan safeguards your assets and spells out your final intentions. It can also help to limit the aging effect on you, ensuring that your wishes are respected and your financial security is maintained throughout your golden years.

The advantages of this plan are that your preferences will be honored, and your financial stability will be preserved. It can help to limit the aging effect on the elderly by protecting their assets and providing clarity for their wishes.

An estate plan can help ensure that the elderly have access to the financial resources they need for their later years. It can also guide decision-making and help to provide clarity in the event of any disputes that may arise with family members or other beneficiaries.

It can also help to limit the aging effect on the elderly by ensuring that their wishes are respected. Making clear decisions about your wishes while you are still alive and in good health can help limit the potential for disputes after you pass away.

It might be challenging to draft an estate plan. While ensuring your wishes are honored, and your financial stability is upheld.

Here are some steps to create an effective estate plan:

1. **Make a list of your assets**: This will help you ensure that all of your assets are accounted for and that you know exactly what you are leaving behind.

2. **Determine who will receive your assets**: It is important to carefully consider who you want to receive your assets and how you want them distributed.

3. **Create documents to formalize your wishes:** You may need to create a will, trust, or other legal documents to fulfill your wishes.

4. **Make sure your documents are up to date**: This is important to ensure your assets are distributed according to your wishes.

MAKING FUNERAL AND BURIAL ARRANGEMENTS

The importance of funeral and burial arrangements cannot be stressed enough before one departs. It can help alleviate some of the stress associated with planning a funeral after a loved one's death, but it can also help limit the aging effect on the elderly.

Making funeral and burial arrangements before a person's passing can help limit the aging effect on the elderly in several ways.

For starters, it takes the burden of making difficult decisions off the shoulders of the surviving family members. This can be especially helpful for the aged, who may be unable to make decisions due to age or frailty. Also, making funeral and burial arrangements before one departs can help reduce the financial strain of a funeral.

A pre-arranged funeral can help to ensure that the financial burden is taken care of in advance so that the family is not stuck with the financial responsibility.

Finally, making funeral and burial arrangements before one departs is beneficial for the elderly as it can help ensure their final wishes are respected and fulfilled. This can be incredibly comforting to the elderly, who may be concerned about not having the opportunity to express their wishes before they pass away.

Now that you understand the importance of making funeral and burial arrangements before one departs, here are some pointers to get you going:

1. **Talk to your family**: Before you begin making arrangements, make sure to talk to your family and let them know what you want. This will ensure that your final wishes are respected and will help to alleviate any stress or confusion for your family.

2. **Make a budget**: Take the time to create a budget for the funeral and burial arrangements. This will help you to determine how much money you can allocate to the funeral and burial and will help you to ensure that you don't overspend.

3. **Research your options**: Take the time to research your options for the funeral and burial arrangements. Consider different venues and pricing options to ensure you get the best deal possible.

4. **Choose a funeral home**: Once you have a budget and have researched, it's time to choose a funeral home. Make sure to choose a reputable funeral home that respects your wishes.

5. **Make arrangements**: Once you have chosen a funeral home, you can begin to make the arrangements. Ensure you include all the details you want, such as music, flowers, and other services.

By taking the time to make funeral and burial arrangements before one departs, you ensure that your final wishes are respected. It can also help alleviate the stress and burden of funeral planning after a loved one's death.

Following the tips mentioned above, you may make the process as easy and stress-free as possible.

DOWNSIZING AND SIMPLIFYING LIFE

I was always busy, running around trying to get things done. I felt like I always had to do something and that I needed to have it all. I was constantly running around and felt like my life was getting out of control.

I was starting to feel the effects of aging, and my body was beginning to show signs of wear and tear. I decided to simplify my life and downsize at that point. I realized I was trying to do too much, which was taking a toll on me.

So, I started to make some changes. I got rid of things I didn't need, cut down on the number of activities I was doing, and began prioritizing my life. I started focusing on the things that mattered to me and stopped worrying about the little things. I began to look at life differently, and I started to enjoy the simple things. I stopped worrying about the future and began to focus on the present.

As I downsized and simplified my life, I noticed something amazing happening. I started to feel younger and healthier. I had more energy and felt like I could do anything. I was sleeping better and feeling more relaxed. I had a sense of regaining control over my life.

As I started to downsize and simplify my life, I also noticed the effects on my body. I felt like I was aging slower and had fewer aches and pains. I felt like I was taking better care of myself and happier and healthier than ever.

Downsizing and simplifying my life have helped me overcome and limit my aging effect. I realized I don't need to have everything and that life is about enjoying the little things. By taking control of my life and focusing on the things that matter most, I'm living the life I was meant to live.

Downsizing and simplifying life can be an important part of helping the elderly to stay healthy and active as they age. It is important to remember that with age comes a need to change our lifestyle and living arrangements to remain independent, healthy, and safe.

It can help to reduce stress, keep up with financial obligations and maintain an active lifestyle. It can also help to reduce clutter, which can be a source of frustration and stress for many people. It limits the impact of aging on the elderly by providing them with a more manageable lifestyle.

The first step in downsizing and simplifying life is to assess your current situation. This can involve evaluating living arrangements, financial obligations, and lifestyle. It is important to determine what is needed and what is not for a comfortable and healthy lifestyle.

Once you have identified your needs and what is no longer needed, the next step is to make changes to your living arrangements and lifestyle. This could involve moving to a smaller home or apartment, reducing your financial obligations, or changing your daily schedule. Depending on your situation, downsizing and simplifying your lifestyle could mean various things.

One way to simplify life is to focus on what is most important to you. This could include spending more time with family and friends, participating in hobbies and activities, or focusing on your health. It is also essential to prioritize your daily tasks and activities, as this can help to reduce stress and prevent burnout.

Downsizing and simplifying life can also involve making changes to your possessions. This could include selling or donating items you no longer need or use. It is also important to keep what is necessary and declutter your home and belongings. This can help to reduce stress, as it eliminates the clutter that can be overwhelming and distracting.

Finally, it is important to remember that downsizing and simplifying life can help to limit the impact of aging on the elderly. It can make life more manageable and easier to keep up with and provide a sense of security, independence, and dignity. It can also help reduce stress, which is essential for maintaining health and well-being.

PREPARING FOR LONG-TERM CARE

A growing number of us are thinking about long-term care as we age. Long-term care provides medical, social, and other support services to people who cannot care for themselves due to age, disability, or other chronic health conditions. It can be provided in various settings, including nursing homes, assisted living facilities, and private residences.

When preparing for long-term care, it's essential to understand that it's not just about providing physical care. It's also about providing emotional and psychological support and helping our elderly loved ones to stay as independent and self-sufficient as possible.

Here are some tips for preparing for long-term care and how it can help to limit the aging effect on the elderly:

1. **Start planning early**: It's important to begin planning for long-term care as soon as possible. The sooner you get started, the more time you'll have to

learn about your alternatives, weigh your options, and make crucial financial and legal decisions.

2. **Consider your needs**: When planning for long-term care, it's essential to consider your needs. Factors to consider may include your current level of health and functional abilities and your emotional needs.

3. **Know your wishes**: It's crucial that you know your long-term care preferences. You may have preferences about the type of care you receive, where you receive it, and who provides it.

4. **Research your options**: Once you know your wishes, it's time to start researching your options. Consider the different types of long-term care available and the cost of each option.

5. **Make a financial plan**: Long-term care can be expensive, so it's essential to make a financial plan to pay for it. Consider the cost of care, and look into potential sources of financial assistance.

6. **Consider legal documents**: It's important to ensure that legal documents are in order so your

wishes are clear. Consider preparing a power of attorney, will, or advance directive.

7. **Find support**: Finding support during this time is important. Look for support groups, counseling services, and other resources to help you on this journey.

Preparing for long-term care can be a difficult and emotional process. However, to ensure that your desires are honored and care is given in the best manner possible, it is crucial to take the time to plan ahead. By understanding the options available and taking the time to make a plan, you can help limit the aging effect and maintain your independence as much as possible.

PROTECTING FINANCES AND ASSETS

As we age, it is important to protect our finances and assets. The aging process can affect our financial security and ability to maintain our lifestyle. By taking proactive steps to protect our finances and assets, we can help limit the impact of aging and ensure our financial security in later life.

Firstly, it is vital to have a financial plan. A financial plan is an important tool for helping to protect and secure our finances.

A good financial plan should include a budget, savings goals, investment strategies, and retirement plans. With a financial plan, you can ensure your finances are secure and manage your money effectively.

Secondly, it is important to protect your assets. You can do this by taking out insurance on your assets, such as your home, car, and other valuable possessions. This will help to ensure that your assets are protected during an unexpected event.

The proper storage of your valuables is another crucial consideration. Consider putting your assets into trusts to protect them from creditors, taxation, and other risks.

Thirdly, it is essential to be aware of scams and fraud. Elderly people are often targeted by scammers looking to exploit their lack of knowledge and experience. Before investing in any financial product or service, do your research. You should also avoid giving anyone personal or financial information over the phone or online.

Finally, it is essential to be aware of your rights. Make sure you understand the laws and regulations pertaining to financial matters, and make sure that you have access to the right information if something goes wrong.

You should also be aware of any scams or frauds targeting elderly individuals and take the necessary steps to protect yourself.

Here are a few types of scams targeted at the elderly:

1. **Phishing**: This type of scam involves sending an email or website link that appears to be from a legitimate source but is actually from a malicious sender. The scammer will often ask for personal information such as credit card numbers and passwords or for the user to click a link that downloads malicious software onto their computer.

2. **Grandparent Scam**: In this type of scam, a scammer will pretend to be a grandchild or other relative of the elderly person and ask them to wire money or send gift cards as a way of helping them out of a financial emergency.

3. **Investment Scams**: These scams target elderly individuals by offering them high-return investment opportunities that are too good to be true. Scammers may use manipulative tactics to get elderly people to invest in fraudulent schemes or projects that don't exist.

4. **Robocall Scams**: Robocalls are automated phone calls that deliver pre-recorded messages. Scammers use these calls to target elderly individuals, often offering them too-good-to-be-true deals or asking for personal information such as Social Security numbers.

5. **Funeral and Cemetery Scams**: These scams target elderly individuals who have recently lost a loved one. Scammers will offer the goods or services related to the funeral or cemetery, such as caskets or grave markers, at inflated prices.

You can protect your finances and possessions and lessen the effects of aging by following the measures mentioned above. With a financial plan, the right insurance, and an awareness of scams and fraud, you can ensure your finances and assets are secure later in life.

CHAPTER 8

AGING GRACEFULLY AND WITH DIGNITY

Aging gracefully and with dignity can be a challenging task, especially if you are not used to the changes that will take place in your body and mind as you grow older. However, with the right attitude, you can make the most of the journey and learn to accept and embrace the process of aging.

The first step in aging gracefully and with dignity is to accept that you are growing older. There is no one-size-fits-all technique for aging, and you must remember that everyone ages differently. It is important to understand that your body and mind will change with time, and you should embrace these changes as part of the natural process of life.

The second step is to take care of your physical and mental health. As you age, your body needs extra care and attention. Exercise regularly, eat a balanced diet, get plenty of rest, and take time to do activities that you enjoy. Also, your mental health needs special attention. Keep in touch with loved ones, express thanks, and partake in joyous and meaningful pursuits.

The third step is to build a strong social network. As you age, staying connected with friends and family is important. You can also join social groups or clubs dedicated to helping older adults stay engaged and connected. These activities can provide much-needed social interaction and a sense of purpose and belonging.

The fourth step is to stay active and engaged. Find activities that are meaningful to you and that you enjoy. This could be anything from taking a class to volunteering in the community. Staying engaged and active will help to keep your mind and body sharp.

The fifth step is to limit the aging effect on your body and mind. One may choose a healthy lifestyle with regular exercise and a well-balanced diet to achieve this. It could also entail taking vitamins and supplements to boost your well-being and health. Additionally, many anti-aging treatments, such as Botox and facial fillers, can help reduce the signs of aging.

Finally, it is important to remember that aging gracefully and with dignity is a journey. You should take daily steps to ensure you lead a purposeful and happy life. Keeping your independence, honor, and a sense of purpose as you age would be helpful.

Aging gracefully and with dignity can be challenging, but it is possible. Taking the time to accept and embrace the changes that come with age, taking care of your physical and mental health, building a strong social network, staying active and engaged, and taking steps to limit the aging effect on your body and mind can all help to make the journey easier. With the right attitude and approach, you can make the most of the journey and age gracefully and with dignity.

STAYING ACTIVE AND ENGAGED

It was a typical day at the hospital, and I was getting ready to see my next patient. I had been a medical doctor for over twenty years and was well-known for my dedication to my patients and commitment to providing the best medical care possible. I have always been active and updated myself with the latest medical technologies and treatments.

I constantly engaged with my patients, asking questions and providing advice and guidance. I enjoyed talking to them and helping them find solutions to their problems. As I got older, I was concerned that I couldn't keep up with my profession's demands as I aged. However, I was determined to stay active and engaged in my work.

I continued to attend medical conferences and seminars, read medical journals and books, and kept in touch with the latest medical developments. I also got plenty of physical exercises, which helped me maintain my energy levels and keep my body in top condition.

Thanks to my activeness and engagement as a medical doctor, I was able to limit the effect of aging on my body and mind. My patients continued to benefit from my expertise and knowledge, and I was able to continue providing them with the highest levels of care. The years passed, and I am still in good health and feeling great. I am grateful for my dedication to my profession and its positive impact on my life.

I realized that my activeness and engagement as a medical doctor enabled me to stay young at heart and enjoy the fruits of my labor for many years.

One thing you can do to maintain good health and vigor as you age is to keep yourself involved and active. It helps to limit the effects of aging on you by keeping the body, mind, and spirit engaged in activities that have been proven to help maintain physical and mental health.

The benefits of staying active and engaged are many. Exercise helps to keep your body strong and improves your balance and coordination, helps to maintain healthy blood pressure, improves your sleep, and even boosts your mood. It can also reduce the risk of diseases like diabetes, stroke, heart disease, and osteoporosis.

Mental engagement is also key to staying active and engaged. Learning new things, challenging yourself, and engaging with others in activities can help to keep your mind sharp, which can help to ward off age-related cognitive decline. Participating in activities you enjoy, such as reading, playing cards, or puzzles, can also help keep your mind active.

Social engagement is another critical component of staying active and engaged. Spending time with loved ones can lift your spirits, ease tension, and offer emotional support. Keeping in touch with those you care about can also help to reduce social isolation, which can be a major factor in age-related decline.

Staying active and engaged will help enrich your life. Participating in activities you enjoy can provide a sense of purpose and meaning, which can help keep you young and happy. From going for walks to taking up a new hobby, there are many ways to stay engaged and active as you age.

Staying active and engaged is essential to keeping yourself healthy and youthful as you age. It helps to limit the effects of aging by keeping the body, mind, and spirit engaged in activities that have been proven to help maintain physical and mental health. So take the time to stay active and engaged, and you'll reap the rewards now and in the years to come.

PURSUING PERSONAL INTERESTS AND HOBBIES

I have a heart for my patients, and I noticed that as they aged, many felt that they were slowly fading away. One day, I decided to take a different approach to help them. I told my patients that instead of focusing on the inevitability of aging, they should focus on pursuing their interests and hobbies. I assured them that although age takes away some of their physical abilities, it can never take away the joy and satisfaction of engaging in a meaningful activity they love.

This approach had an immediate and positive impact on them. They began to feel invigorated and motivated to try out new things. I watched them grow in confidence as they become more engaged in activities they enjoyed. I became proud of them for taking the initiative to pursue activities that made them happy. They were living life to the fullest and embracing the aging process. I am filled with joy to see that my advice has helped my patients limit the effects of aging by finding purpose and joy in the activities they choose to pursue.

Pursuing personal interests and hobbies is a great way to keep your body active and your mind sharp as you age. Also, it can aid in reducing stress and promoting social connection, both of which are essential components of healthy aging.

People often think of hobbies as something only children do, but they can be just as beneficial for adults. Hobbies can help keep us mentally, emotionally, and physically active, providing a much-needed break from the daily grind of life. They can also help us to stay connected to our creativity, which can help us to keep our minds active and alert.

For elders, pursuing personal interests and hobbies can provide an escape from the monotony of day-to-day life, offer a sense of accomplishment, and help reduce stress. Many find that engaging in activities they enjoy can be a great way to prevent boredom, keep their minds active, and help them stay social.

Activities such as gardening, painting, writing, or playing a musical instrument can provide a great source of relaxation and help reduce stress.

Participating in physical activities like yoga, swimming, or walking can also help to maintain physical fitness and well-being. For elders who may not have the mobility or physical abilities to participate in active hobbies, many activities can be done seated or with the help of a caregiver. These include reading, playing card or board games, or conversing with friends or family.

Pursuing personal interests and hobbies can also allow you to share your knowledge and experience with others. For example, some of you may teach classes about your hobbies, such as knitting, cooking, or woodworking. This can be a great way to stay connected with the community, meet new people, and help to pass on valuable knowledge.

Following one's passions and hobbies can help slow down the consequences of aging in addition to the physical and mental advantages. This is because hobbies can help to give you a sense of purpose and can help to combat loneliness and depression, which can be common in the elderly. Participating in activities you enjoy is a wonderful way to stay in shape as you age and lessen the consequences of aging.

Hence, if you're looking for a means to continue being engaged, try pursuing a hobby or two – you'll be glad you did!

MAINTAINING INDEPENDENCE

As we age, many challenges arise. Many of us struggle to maintain independence, especially when we become elderly. But maintaining our independence is important to age well and live a healthy life. It can help limit the effects of aging and give us more control over our lives.

In this chapter, we will discuss the importance of maintaining independence and how it can help us to overcome the effects of aging.

The first step in maintaining independence is to stay active. Exercise helps to keep muscles strong, improve balance, and prevent the onset of illnesses that can reduce mobility and independence. Finding a recreational activity that fits your age and physical capabilities is fundamental. If needed, seek the help of a physical therapist or trainer to help you find a safe and suitable exercise routine.

The second step is to stay connected with friends and family. Social interaction is essential for mental and emotional well-being. Stay in touch with friends and family, both in person and online. This can help you stay engaged and connected to the world.

Next, stay active mentally. Keeping your mind active and engaged can help to ward off mental decline. Read, take classes, play games, and pursue challenging hobbies. By actively engaging your mind, you can help to reduce the effects of aging on the brain.

Finally, stay independent financially. Having a secure financial plan to remain independent as you age is important. This includes planning for retirement and setting up a budget that you can stick to.

Staying active and engaged in life, both physically and mentally, is essential to living a whole and independent life. By following these steps, you can help to ensure that you remain independent and active as you age.

Benefits of Maintaining Independence

Maintaining independence as we age can have many benefits. It can help us to stay active and engaged in our life, which can help us to stay healthier. It can also help us to remain independent longer, as independence can help us to manage our medical needs, keep up with our social obligations, and stay connected with our community.

For the elderly, maintaining independence can also help to limit the effects of aging. Falling can be dangerous for elders' health and can be reduced by doing this. It can also help to reduce the risk of depression, anxiety, and other mental health issues that can come with aging.

Finally, it can help improve our overall quality of life and give us more control over our lives.

How to Maintain Independence

Maintaining independence as we age is important but can also be challenging. The following tips will assist you in preserving your independence as you get older:

- **Start budgeting and planning for your future**: Making a budget and planning for your future will help you become independent as you age.

Figure out how much money you need to support yourself and how you can save for retirement.

- **Live within your means**: Try to limit your spending and save as much as possible for the future. This will help you become more independent and secure in your finances.

- **Start investing**: Investing your money can help you become financially independent and secure long-term. Consider different types of investments, such as stocks, bonds, mutual funds, and ETFs.

- **Build your credit**: Building good credit is essential for becoming independent. Make sure you make all payments on time and pay off any debt quickly.

- **Create an emergency fund**: An emergency fund can help you stay independent when unexpected expenses arise. Consider setting aside some money each month to build up your emergency fund.

- **Seek financial advice**: Talking to a financial advisor can help you become more financially independent. They can help you create a strategy

and provide advice on investments, budgeting, and
more.

- **Create a retirement plan**: Creating a retirement
plan early on can help you become independent
when you're older. Consider different types of
retirement savings accounts, such as an IRA or
401(k).
- **Take care of your health**: Taking care of your
health is essential for remaining independent. Make
sure to eat healthily, exercise regularly, and get
enough sleep.

- **Stay socially active**: Staying socially active can
help to keep you connected with your friends and
family, which can help to maintain your
independence.

- **Stay organized**: Staying organized can help you
take the necessary steps to maintain your
independence.

- **Take care of your mental health**. Maintaining
good mental health can lower your risk of developing
depression and other mental health problems.

Overall, maintaining independence as one ages is essential to limiting the effect of aging. Regular physical, intellectual, and social activities can help to reduce the physical and mental effects of aging while promoting a sense of control, autonomy, and self-confidence.

CELEBRATING LIFE ACCOMPLISHMENT

Celebrating life accomplishments is an important part of aging with grace. It is an effective way to keep growing and experiencing life meaningfully. As we age, we naturally become more introspective and reflect on our accomplishments and failures.

Celebrating our accomplishments can be a great way to counter the effects of aging. The first thing to understand is that age has nothing to do with our accomplishments. So, when we celebrate our life accomplishments, we are not celebrating our age. We are celebrating our achievements and lessons learned along the way. This helps us recognize that life is about learning and growing, regardless of age.

Second, when we celebrate our life accomplishments, we can find strength in the memories of our past successes. This can give us the motivation to go on and continue to strive for new experiences and to create new goals. It can remind us that we still have much to offer in the present and future.

Third, when we celebrate our life accomplishments, we can recognize and appreciate the effort and time we have put into each accomplishment. Taking time to be proud of ourselves helps build self-confidence and self-esteem. This can help to keep us feeling young and vibrant.

Celebrating our accomplishments can be a great way to stay connected with family and friends. Sharing our experiences and stories can help keep us connected and part of a larger community. It also provides a way to keep our memory alive and to share our life's journey with others.

As I approach retirement, I reflect on my life and feel a sense of accomplishment for everything I have achieved. I have made a difference in countless people's lives through my work. Celebrating my life accomplishments has helped curb the effects of aging as I grow old.

My aspirations for my future were clear when I was younger and after seeing how my dynamic mother became frail with age. I wanted to be a doctor who could help people and positively impact the world. My dreams were realized when I graduated from medical school and began my journey as a medical doctor.

Through my work, I saved lives, comforted those suffering, and helped people understand preventive care's importance. As I get older, my accomplishments as a doctor have taken on an even greater significance.

By celebrating the successes of my career, I can focus on the positive and stay motivated to keep making a difference. I am also reminded of the importance of caring for myself and my body to ensure I remain healthy and can continue helping those in need.

By celebrating my successes and the impact I have made in the lives of others, I am able to feel a sense of accomplishment and pride in my work. This helps to keep me motivated and feeling young as I age. I am also reminded of the importance of taking care of myself and my body so that I can continue to help those in need.

My life, in general, has been filled with accomplishments, and I am proud to reflect on it. As I get older, celebrating my accomplishments has helped me slow down the effects of aging, and I am grateful for everything I have accomplished in my life.

You can celebrate your life accomplish by doing the following:

1. **Throw a Party**: Throwing a party is a great way for you to celebrate life's accomplishments. Invite family, friends, and neighbors to join in the celebration. Ask everyone to bring a dish to share, decorate the home, and provide a few games or activities. Be sure to include some of your favorite foods and music.

2. **Take a Trip**: Taking a trip is a great way for you to celebrate life's accomplishments. Choose a meaningful destination, such as an area you lived in when you were younger, a family vacation spot, or somewhere you have always wanted to visit. Make sure to plan activities suitable for your physical condition.

3. **Create a Memory Book**: Create a memory book to commemorate accomplishments. Include photos, mementos, and stories from your personal life. Ask family and friends to contribute their memories and stories. This will be a great way for you to reflect on the wonderful things you have achieved throughout your lifetime.

4. **Make a Video**: Make a video of you talking about your life accomplishments. Share stories and photos from your life. This can be a great way to document and share your accomplishments with family and friends.

5. **Hold a Presentation**: Hold a presentation to honor your life accomplishments. Invite family, friends, and neighbors to attend. Present mementos and photos to share. Provide refreshments and a few activities. This will be a great way of recognizing you and your accomplishments.

LIVING WITH JOY AND HAPPINESS

There's this seventy-year-old man with chronic pain and illness for the past fifteen years. He was diagnosed with osteoarthritis in his knees, diabetes, and high blood pressure. He was taking numerous medications, was limited in physical activity, and became increasingly isolated from his friends and family. He had become depressed and was constantly in a state of misery.

One day, He had a conversation with me about his health, and I suggested that one way to improve his condition was to focus on living with joy and happiness. The gentleman was initially skeptical, but he decided to try it. He started by making small changes in his daily life. He began taking short walks outside and appreciating the beauty of nature.

He also started listening to music and reading books that inspired him. He set up a daily routine with light exercises, meditation, and yoga. He also began to make an effort to connect with people consciously. He reached out to old friends and family members whom he hadn't spoken to in a while and spent quality time with them. He started attending social gatherings and events and made a point of being generous and kind to others.

The gentleman noticed that these small changes he was making to his life positively impacted his health. His pain and other symptoms began to diminish, and he started to feel more energetic. He was also more engaged in his social life and felt more connected to the people around him.

After a couple of months, I was amazed by the improvement in his health. I was so impressed that I recommended his story to other patients struggling with chronic illnesses. After seeing the results of his efforts, they, too, began to make positive changes in their lives and started to see improvements in their health.

His story is an inspiring example of how living with joy and happiness can tremendously impact our health. By making small changes to his lifestyle and connecting with the people around him, he reduced his chronic pain and improved his overall health. His story inspires us all to take care of our health and make the most of each day we have.

Living with joy and happiness is something that everyone should strive for in life, especially as we get older. Our bodies and minds change as we age, but that doesn't mean we can't live joyful lives. The key is to focus on the things that bring us joy and happiness and to make sure we take time to appreciate them.

A relationship-centered approach is one of the best ways to add joy and happiness to our lives. Spending time with family and friends is a great way to boost our mood and make us feel appreciated. We should also take time to nurture our relationships by having meaningful conversations, going on fun outings, and showing appreciation for the people in our lives.

We should also take time to appreciate the little things in life. We can do this by engaging in activities that bring us joy, like going for a walk, reading a book, or listening to music. We can also take time to appreciate nature by going for a hike, spending time in a park, or even just sitting and admiring the beauty of the world around us. Taking time to appreciate the little things can help us find joy even in the most difficult times.

Another way to live a life of joy and happiness is to take care of our physical and mental health. This means eating healthy, exercising regularly, getting enough sleep, and managing any stress or anxiety that we may feel. By caring for our bodies and minds, we may slow down the effects of aging and improve our general well-being.

Finally, it is important to remember that joy and happiness come from within. We should focus on what makes us happy and permit ourselves to enjoy life. This could mean taking up a new hobby, learning a new skill, or simply relaxing and unwinding. Taking time to focus on ourselves can help us find joy and happiness in our lives, regardless of age.

Living with joy and happiness is something we should all strive for, especially as we age. Taking time to appreciate our relationships, appreciate the little things in life, take care of our physical and mental health, and focus on what makes us happy can help us limit aging and lead a life of joy and happiness.

CHAPTER 9

SPIRITUAL GROWTH IN OLD AGE

As we age, our spiritual life often takes a back seat to the physical and emotional changes that come with growing old. We tend to focus on physical health, managing finances, and staying connected to family and friends. But it's important to remember that our spiritual growth and well-being can play a huge role in helping us to manage the aging process and limit the effects of aging.

The first step to spiritual growth in old age is recognizing that your spiritual life can be just as vital as your physical or emotional health. Even if you're not religious, you still have a spiritual life. It's your part connected to a higher power, nature, or an inner sense of peace. Your general well-being can be significantly enhanced by making the time to cultivate your spiritual practice.

One of the most important aspects of spiritual growth in old age is to be mindful of the present moment. It can be simple to become mired in concerns about the future or disappointments about the past, but focusing on the now can help you achieve serenity and happiness. It's important to remain conscious of your thoughts and emotions and take the time to appreciate the wonders of nature, the world around you, and the people in your life.

Being mindful of the present moment can also help to reduce stress, which can be a major factor in aging.

Finding a spiritual practice that is meaningful to you is also important. This could be anything from yoga to meditation, prayer, or just spending time in nature. Whatever it is, be sure it resonates with you and brings you comfort. Taking the time for your spiritual practice can help to reduce stress, bring clarity to your thoughts, and help you to feel more connected to the world around you.

Finally, it's important to be kind to yourself. As we age, it's easy to focus on all the things we can't do or can't control, but it's important to recognize that you are still capable of so much. Take the time to appreciate yourself, your strengths, and your weaknesses, and be gentle with yourself. Recognize your accomplishments and the journey you've been on, and remember that you can still grow and improve. Spiritual growth in old age can be a powerful tool in helping to manage the aging process and limit the effects of aging. You can make the most of your remaining years by recognizing the importance of your spiritual life, being mindful of the present moment, finding a meaningful spiritual practice, and being kind to yourself.

CULTIVATING A SPIRIT OF GRATITUDE

Gratitude has been a life-changing practice for me. It has helped me become a more positive and self-aware individual who can better accept and appreciate life's blessings. I have benefited immensely from the practice of gratitude, not just at this stage of my life but throughout my life.

Gratitude has helped me recognize the positive aspects of my life and to appreciate the good things that come my way. It has allowed me to be more mindful of the blessings and joys in my life and better express my appreciation for them.

Expressing gratitude has also helped me develop a deeper connection with myself and those around me. It has allowed me to recognize better and be more grateful for my life's blessings. At my age, I have found that gratitude has helped me to manage my emotions better and to remain positive in the face of challenges. It has helped me to focus on the present moment and to be more content with what I have. Gratitude has also helped me remain resilient in the face of difficult circumstances and thankful for the good things that come my way.

Overall, I have benefited immensely from the practice of gratitude in my old age. It has helped me stay positive, be more content with what I have, and remain thankful for the blessings in my life. I am very grateful for the practice of gratitude, which has made my old age a much more enjoyable and fulfilling experience.

As we age, it's easy to become consumed by our aches, pains, and the body's physical limitations. But cultivating a spirit of gratitude can make a big difference if you want to limit the effects of aging. A spirit of gratitude is an attitude of thankfulness and appreciation for all the good in your life. It's a reminder that while age may change your body, it doesn't have to affect your attitude and outlook.

Benefits of Cultivating a Spirit of Gratitude

Cultivating a spirit of gratitude can help you in several ways. Gratitude has been linked to greater physical, mental, and emotional well-being. It can improve mood, reduce stress, and increase overall happiness. Also, it can foster a more positive outlook on life, which in turn can help limit the effects of aging.

The Power of Gratitude

Gratitude can change our thoughts, feelings, and behaviors. It can give us a new perspective and help us see the positive in difficult times. Rather than dwelling on our losses, we can focus on the things we still have. We can find joy in simple pleasures and appreciate even the smallest blessings.

Practicing gratitude

The best way to cultivate a spirit of gratitude is to practice it daily. To get you started, consider these tips:

• Take time each day to think about all the good things in your life.

• Write a gratitude journal, noting everything you are thankful for.

• Appreciate those who have influenced your life and tell them how grateful you are.

• Say "thank you" more frequently till it becomes a habit.

• Make an effort to count your blessings each day.

• Give back to your community in some way.

• Show appreciation for even the smallest of things.

Embracing an attitude of appreciation can slow down the effects of aging. It can elevate mood, lessen stress, and boost general contentment. Daily gratitude exercises help us recognize even the tiniest blessings and delight in everyday activities. So, count your blessings and be thankful for all the good in your life.

FINDING INNER PEACE

Finding inner peace is a lifelong journey that can benefit people of all ages, but it can be especially beneficial for older adults. After all, aging can bring about many physical, mental, and emotional changes, many of which can be challenging to cope with.

It is imperative than ever to preserve our inner peace and balance as we age if we want to be healthy and enjoy life. In this chapter, I'll explore how finding inner peace can help limit the aging effect on older people, and I'll also discuss some practical ways to cultivate inner peace and balance.

To bring the concepts to life, I'll also include a captivating story about a woman who found inner peace and a new purpose in life despite her advanced age.

Hazel was a vibrant and energetic woman in her late seventies. Despite her age, she was still actively involved in her community, volunteering at the local library and socializing with her loved ones. But then, her life changed abruptly when her husband passed away. She was devastated and felt like her entire world had been turned upside down. She was overwhelmed with grief and felt like she had no purpose in life anymore.

At first, she tried to cope with her grief by distracting herself. She kept busy with her volunteer work, but it only brought her temporary relief. It's clear to her that she needed to find a way to cope with her grief and find a new purpose in life. That's when Hazel decided to take up yoga and meditation. She had heard that these practices could help her find inner peace and was willing to try them.

At first, she was a bit skeptical, but she was soon amazed by its profound effect on her. Through yoga and meditation, Hazel was able to connect with her inner self and find a sense of peace and balance. She also discovered a new purpose in life; she wanted to share her newfound inner peace with others and help them find their inner balance.

Hazel began teaching yoga and meditation classes to other elders in her community. Soon, she inspired others to find inner peace and balance. She felt fulfilled and amazed at how much younger she felt.

The Benefits of Finding Inner Peace

Hazel's story illustrates the incredible benefits of finding inner peace. Let's look at some ways it can help limit the aging effect on you.

First, inner peace can help reduce stress and anxiety. As we age, it's common to experience increased stress and anxiety levels due to physical, mental, and emotional changes. But cultivating inner peace can help reduce stress and anxiety and make coping with life's challenges easier.

Second, inner peace can boost mental clarity and focus. As we age, it's common to experience mental clarity and focus declines. But by cultivating inner peace, we can boost our mental clarity and focus and enjoy a sharper, more alert mind.

Third, inner peace can help maintain physical health. Our physical health tends to decline as we age due to body changes. But cultivating inner peace can help keep our bodies in balance and reduce the physical effects of aging.

Fourth, inner peace can help us maintain a positive attitude. As we age, it's common to experience depression, anxiety, and low self-esteem. But cultivating inner peace can help us maintain a positive attitude and enjoy a more fulfilling life.

Finally, inner peace can help us find a renewed sense of purpose. As we age, finding a sense of purpose and meaning in life can be difficult. But cultivating inner peace can help us find a renewed purpose and enjoy our golden years.

How to Cultivate Inner Peace

Let's look at some practical ways to cultivate inner peace now that we know its benefits. First, practice mindfulness.

First, practice mindfulness. Being mindful is paying attention to our thoughts and feelings as they arise in the present moment without passing judgment. It can help us be more aware of our inner self and cultivate inner peace.

Second, take time for yourself. Taking time out of your day is important to focus on yourself and your needs. This could include activities such as meditating, exercising, or simply taking a walk in nature.

Third, practice self-care. Self-care is taking care of your physical, mental, and emotional needs. It could include getting enough sleep, eating a healthy diet, and engaging in activities that bring you joy.

Fourth, practice gratitude. Taking time to appreciate what we are grateful for can help us cultivate inner peace and balance.

Finally, connect with others. Connecting with others is an important part of finding inner peace. It can help us feel connected, loved, and supported.

Finding inner peace is important to stay healthy and enjoy life as we age. It can help us reduce stress and anxiety, boost mental clarity and focus, maintain physical health, maintain a positive attitude, and find a renewed sense of purpose. In addition to the practical tips outlined in this chapter, Hazel's story illustrates the powerful effects of finding inner peace. Her story is a reminder that it's never too late to find inner peace and a new purpose in life.

CULTIVATING A SENSE OF PURPOSE

As we age, it can be difficult to maintain the same energy and enthusiasm as we were younger. We may find that life's challenges become more difficult to manage and that our minds and bodies don't respond similarly. But there is hope. The aging effect on you can be overcome and limited by developing a sense of purpose.

I remember watching my mother grow old and frail. She was always dynamic and energetic, but I saw her slowly change as she aged. She became less active, and her enthusiasm for life seemed to fade. Watching the woman who had always been my source of strength and support become increasingly dependent on others was heartbreaking. But it wasn't all bad.

Despite her physical limitations, my mother continued to find joy and purpose in life. She found ways to engage with the world around her, explore her interests, and stay connected with friends and family. Her sense of purpose kept her going, allowing her to feel fulfilled in life and makes the most of her later years.

Cultivating a sense of purpose at any age is possible, even as we grow older. To get you started, consider the following recommendation:

• **Identify Your Interests**: Consider what interests you and how you would like to spend your time. Maybe it's writing, crafting, or chatting with friends. Perhaps it's traveling or exploring the outdoors. Whatever it is, make sure it brings you joy and a feeling of accomplishment.

• Find Ways to Engage: Once you've identified your interests, find ways to engage in them. This could include taking classes, volunteering, or participating in activities with others. It's important to stay connected to the world and find ways to contribute.

• **Take Care of Yourself**: Make sure you care for yourself physically and mentally. Eat a balanced diet, stay active, and get enough rest. Caring for your body and mind will help you stay energized and motivated.

• **Live Each Day to the Fullest**: Make the most of each day. Find joy in the little things, be grateful for the blessings in your life, and find ways to make a difference. Don't take life for granted – take the time to appreciate all you have.

We can combat and mitigate the effects of aging by developing a sense of purpose. It can give us energy, enthusiasm, and motivation to live life to the fullest. We can make the most of our later years by engaging in activities that bring us joy, taking care of ourselves, and living each day to the fullest.

CONNECTING WITH HIGHER POWER

In today's world, aging is unavoidable. As we approach our twilight years, many feel that their best days are behind them and that their life is coming to an end. Nevertheless, this is not a need. Research has shown that connecting with higher power can help overcome and limit the aging effect on the elderly, promoting physical and mental health, mental clarity, and a sense of purpose. When it comes to aging, it's not always about physical changes.

As we age, our mental health can suffer, leading to feelings of anxiety, depression, and loneliness. Connecting with a higher power allows us to find solace and peace as we age. Connecting with higher power can provide us with an anchor in our lives, a source of strength that can help us cope with the stresses of aging and the changes that come with it.

The positive effects of connecting with higher power can be seen in numerous ways. Studies have found that elderly individuals with a strong spiritual or religious belief system experience better mental health and well-being than those without. They are also more likely to have healthy relationships with others and have a greater sense of purpose. Connecting with a higher power can also help us to find meaning and joy in our lives, even as we age.

The benefits of connecting with a higher power can be further enhanced when combined with other forms of self-care. Exercise, healthy eating, and socializing are all important parts of maintaining physical and mental health as we age.

Additionally, engaging in activities such as journaling, meditation, and prayer can help us to find peace and connection with our spiritual side.

Mr. Smith was an elderly man of eighty-five years old. He had lived a whole life but had recently been feeling the effects of age. He was lonely, anxious, and had lost his sense of purpose. Though he did not consider himself a spiritual person, he decided to try connecting with a higher power and began praying every day. At first, he found it difficult to focus on his prayers. He felt disconnected and struggled to find the words to express himself. But over time, he discovered that connecting with a higher power filled him with peace and calm.

He began to feel more connected to others, and his sense of purpose was restored. Mr. Smith also found that connecting with a higher power helped him to manage the physical and mental effects of aging. He was able to accept the changes that come with age and found joy in the little things.

He even began to find comfort in the loneliness he had once feared. Mr. Smith's story is a testament to the power of connecting with a higher power. It is a reminder that even in our twilight years, we can find peace, joy, and purpose in our lives. By connecting with a higher power, we can overcome and limit the aging effect on the elderly, promoting physical and mental health, mental clarity, and a sense of purpose.

CHAPTER 10

CELEBRATING LIFE AND EMBRACING LEGACY

The elderly have many years of life experience and wisdom to share, which can make them invaluable assets to those around them. However, age does not mean the elderly or their legacy must be forgotten. They can remain vital and active in their communities, and by celebrating life and embracing legacy, they can limit the aging effect on their lives.

No one is ever too old to appreciate life and all the beautiful moments it can bring. For the elderly, these moments can be especially valuable, as they provide an opportunity to appreciate all they have accomplished in life and all they still have to look forward to. Celebrating life and embracing legacy can give you a sense of purpose and belonging and help you maintain a positive attitude, regardless of age.

One of the most powerful ways of celebrating life and embracing legacy is by spending time with family and friends, especially those of a similar age and with similar experiences. Spending time with those who understand and appreciate you can help ease the loneliness and stress often accompanying aging. It can also help to keep you connected to your communities, which can be especially beneficial for those who are no longer able to work or attend social events.

My Grandpa was one such elderly man. He had been a hard-working farmer all his life, but as he aged, he had to give up his beloved farm to his children and could no longer work the land. He was devastated and felt like his life was over. But then he started getting together with his friends and neighbors at the local diner and sharing stories of his life, struggles, and successes.

His friends began to look up to him as a source of wisdom and guidance, and they began to make time to visit him. Grandpa was able to find joy in his life again, and his friends were able to appreciate his wisdom and experience. He was able to pass down his knowledge and values to the younger generations, and I still remember the stories my father told me about him. It was a way for him to celebrate life and embrace his legacy.

There are many ways for the elderly to celebrate life and embrace their legacy. Taking up a hobby or getting involved in the community can help the elderly to stay active and engaged. Reading books and keeping up with the latest news can help them to stay informed and connected to the world around them. Spending time with family and friends is another great way to celebrate life and embrace legacy, and it can help to keep the elderly feeling connected and appreciated.

By celebrating life and embracing legacy, you can remain active and engaged members of your community and continue to pass down your wisdom and experience to the younger generations. Through these activities, you can limit the aging effect on your life, allowing you to remain vibrant and engaged.

REFLECTING ON LIFE ACCOMPLISHMENTS

There was an elderly patient who reminded me of my mother when she visited my hospital. She had lived a long and full life but was starting to feel her age. Her joints ached, her energy levels were low, and she was losing her sense of purpose.

After she tabled her complaint before me, since I have dealt with familiar cases in the past, I told her to take a moment and reflect on all the accomplishments she had achieved throughout her life. She thought about all the people she had helped, all the obstacles she had overcome, and all the wonderful moments she had experienced.

As she reminisced, something magical began to happen. She began to feel a renewed sense of vitality and purpose. She realized that despite her age, she still had much to offer the world. This realization invigorated her and gave her newfound energy and optimism.

The power of reflecting on life accomplishments can be extremely beneficial for any elderly person. It can help them overcome the feeling of being useless and powerless; instead, it can make them feel empowered and valued. It can help them shift their focus from their age and limitations to their accomplishments and their positive impact on the world.

By reflecting on your life accomplishments, you can gain a newfound sense of purpose and meaning. You may feel inspired to share your wisdom and stories with younger generations or be motivated to pursue new activities and hobbies. This can be a great way to combat the effects of aging, as it gives you a sense of purpose and value.

Reflecting on life accomplishments can also help you to connect with and appreciate your past. It can help you remember the moments of joy and wonder and recognize your strength and resilience. When you are able to look back on your life, you can take pride in the accomplishments you have achieved and also feel grateful for the experiences you've had.

Reflecting on life accomplishments can be a powerful tool for elderly people to maintain a sense of purpose and meaning. The woman's story is an inspiring example of the power of reflection and how it can help limit the aging effect on the elderly. By reflecting on all your accomplishments, you can gain a newfound sense of vitality, purpose, and appreciation for life.

SHARING STORIES AND WISDOM

Sharing stories and wisdom is one of the best ways to overcome and limit the aging effect on the elderly. It is an effective mechanism that can help to maintain and even improve their mental and physical health.

Stories are powerful tools that allow us to connect with others, share our experiences, and learn from one another. They can provide comfort and understanding, help to bridge generational gaps, and help you feel more connected to the world. When you share your stories, you can reflect on your life and the experiences that shaped you. This reflection can be an incredibly powerful experience, as it can help you remember your personal history and better understand your current life.

Sharing stories can also help you make sense of your life and gain a sense of purpose and meaning.

Older adults can also benefit from sharing their wisdom. This wisdom can be drawn from their life experiences and is a valuable resource for younger generations. Sharing wisdom can help to pass on lessons that have been learned and can provide insight into different aspects of life. It can also help to create a strong sense of community and connection between generations.

When sharing stories and wisdom, it is essential to remember to be respectful and considerate of the elderly. Respect their wishes and their right to privacy, and take the time to listen to what they have to say. Also, it's important to be compassionate, patient, and conscious of their potential physical or mental limits.

Sharing stories and wisdom can be a meaningful experience for the elderly and their families. It can help them feel connected and purposeful while also slowing down the effects of aging. By listening to their stories and wisdom, we can gain insight into the lives of our elderly loved ones and help create a stronger bond between generations.

BUILDING A LEGACY

Many of us feel a sense of helplessness and dread about aging. Whether it's worrying about our physical and mental health or the impact of age on our relationships and finances, it's easy to feel overwhelmed. However, there is one thing that can help us to combat the effects of aging: building a legacy.

Building a legacy is an integral part of life, regardless of our age. It involves creating something that will outlive us, something that others can remember us by. It can range from something small, such as a photo album, to something much bigger, such as a foundation or charity. Whatever it is, building a legacy helps to provide a sense of purpose in life and to ensure that our lives have a lasting impact on the world.

For the elderly, building a legacy can be especially powerful. It provides a way to stay connected to the world and engaged in life, even as physical and mental health decline. It also helps to give them a sense of accomplishment and satisfaction, as they can look back and see how their efforts have contributed to the lives of others.

Building a legacy can also be an effective way to combat the physical effects of aging. By staying engaged with your interests and hobbies, you can stay physically active and keep your mind sharp. By doing so, the chances of contracting age-related disorders like dementia and Alzheimer's can be reduced.

Finally, building a legacy can be a great way to help you retain your independence. By creating something that can be shared with others, you can stay connected to your community and maintain your sense of identity. This can help you to remain socially active and to foster meaningful relationships.

CELEBRATING LIFE AND EMBRACING THE FUTURE

Life is a priceless gift that should be cherished and appreciated, particularly as we age. It is important to recognize the aging process, but with the right attitude and outlook, we can limit the effects of aging and continue to live life to the fullest.

As we age, we are faced with different physical, emotional, and mental changes. It can take time to adjust and accept these changes as part of the aging process. One way to overcome this is to focus on the positives of aging. For example, we can take advantage of the wisdom that comes with age and use it to make wise decisions. We can also appreciate the relationships we have developed over the years and our experiences.

Another way to embrace aging is to stay active and keep our minds and bodies healthy. Exercise is a great way to stay in shape and keep our energy levels high. Eating a balanced diet and getting enough sleep are also important for maintaining physical and mental health. Reading, puzzles, and socializing can also help keep our minds sharp.

Staying positive and focusing on the good in life is also essential. We can practice gratitude and appreciation for the things we have and the experiences we have been through. Practicing mindfulness can also help us stay in touch with our feelings and appreciate the present moment.

Finally, celebrating life and embracing the future can help us overcome the effect of aging and live life to the fullest. We can celebrate our successes and appreciate our accomplishments. We can also focus on achieving our goals and look forward to the future enthusiastically and eagerly.

LIVING WITH GRATITUDE AND HAPPINESS

Living with gratitude and happiness is essential for overcoming and limiting the aging effect on the elderly. As we age, our physical and mental health can decline, making it more difficult to enjoy life as we once did. Fortunately, there are proactive steps we can take to ensure our well-being and reduce the aging effect.

Living with gratitude and happiness can help us to maintain a positive outlook and make the most of our golden years. One way to maintain a positive outlook and enjoy the aging process is to practice gratitude. Being thankful for the life we have can make us appreciate what we have and be content with our current situation.

Gratitude, according to research, can boost general happiness, reduce stress and depression, and enhance physical and psychological health. Keeping a gratitude journal is one approach to cultivating gratitude. Writing down three to five things we are grateful for daily can help us focus on the positive and remind us of the good things in life. We can also practice gratitude by showing appreciation for those around us. Whether expressing our gratitude for our family and friends or taking the time to thank someone for a kind act, it can make us feel more connected and bring more joy into our lives.

Another way to make the most of our golden years is to focus on the present. Living in the moment can help us to enjoy life more fully and appreciate the small moments that make up our days. We can also practice mindfulness, which is being aware of our thoughts and feelings and accepting them without judgment. Mindfulness can help us be more present in our lives and become more aware of our emotions and feelings.

Finally, practicing happiness can help us to stay positive and make the most of our golden years. Happiness is more than a feeling; it's a state of mind. Taking the time to focus on what brings us joy can help us to appreciate the good things in life and stay motivated.

We can also practice self-care and do things that make us feel good, such as exercise, meditate, or take a relaxing bath. With the right attitude and tools, we can make the most of our golden years and enjoy a happy and healthy life.

CONCLUSION

This book provides an insightful and inspiring look into the life of the elderly and those preparing for retirement. It passes a hopeful message that aging need not be a dreaded prospect but can bring a new stage of life to be embraced. It emphasizes that growing old is not the end but an opportunity to discover new passions and experiences. Through the stories of those who have embraced their aging years shared, the book encourages readers to do the same. It also encourages readers to find joy in their lives and to appreciate the experiences they have had.

Key takeaways include growing old is not the final step towards the grave but rather a new chapter of life to be enjoyed and experienced. It is full of hope that with the right outlook and attitude, retirement and the golden years can be a time of growth, exploration, and fulfillment. It also emphasized the importance of staying active, both physically and mentally, as well as maintaining meaningful relationships.

By embracing the changes that come with aging, readers can rest assured that a whole life is to be lived in their golden years.

References

Opthalmology, A. A. (n.d.). Retrieved from
https://www.aao.org/eye-health/diseases/what-is-presbyopia